Improving School Mental Health

Improving School Mental Health

The Thriving School Community Solution

Charle Peck

Dr. Cameron Caswell

ConnectEDD Publishing
Hanover, Pennsylvania

This publication is available at discount pricing when purchased in quantity for educational purposes, promotions, or fundraisers. For inquiries and details, contact the publisher at: info@connecteddpublishing.com

Published by ConnectEDD Publishing LLC
Hanover, PA
www.connecteddpublishing.com

Cover Design: Kheila Dunkerly

Improving School Mental Health/ Charle Peck and Cameron Caswell. —1st ed.
Paperback ISBN 979-8-9860690-9-8

ConnectEDD
PUBLISHING

Praise for *Improving School Mental Health*

As an educator, it is easy to feel overwhelmed with different kinds of learners and their varying needs. This resource is set up to be manageable, actionable shifts a teacher can make that don't make more work in the planning and preparation side of teaching. As a parent, the resource has helped me recognize some of the reactive behaviors I exhibit and has given me some tools of self-reflection that I can use at home and in the classroom. The analogies used in the book help the reader connect easily to the situation that is being presented, and the "Biggest Takeaways" make it easy for stakeholders to quickly refer back to the resource. This book should be on any guardian or teachers' must-read list; it is the resource we need to transform youth mental health.

—Nicole Gerbes | Student Success Teacher (9-12) and parent

Improving School Mental Health is a game changer for helping our students and teachers where they need it most! This book is full of relatable examples, and it guides you to utilize what you are already doing. The well-developed tools and strategies help you get to the root cause of the problem, fortify you with rapid resets to help de-escalate the student in the crucial moment, and leads you through practical strategies for long term success. This book lives up to the TSC mission to energize educators, empower students, and engage parents.

—Kathleen Eckert | Director of Compliance and Policy, Author of
School Transformation Through Teacher Appreciation

The mental health crisis that our young people face today cannot be overstated. In our post pandemic, social media-saturated world, the hearts and minds of our children are more vulnerable than ever before in history. This book offers clear, accessible solutions to address one of the most critical problems of our time. Let's help our kids thrive. Spread this book far and wide.

—Ofosu Jones-Quartey | Author of *Love Your Amazing Self*

If you are serious about improving mental health at your school, you will check out *Improving School Mental Health: The Thriving School Community Solution*. The authors provide real solutions that real schools can implement immediately to help solve one of the biggest challenges facing our schools today. Mental health will be THE issue of the next decade in our schools, and I believe this book will become THE resource schools go to for real answers!

—Pat Quinn | "The RTI Guy" Author of the book *Ultimate RTI*

This is a book that I have needed for years to help change the perspective we take when working with students and balancing their school stress and their mental health. I am so grateful to have a new therapeutic approach to guide my therapy sessions with clients, parents, and the school system, especially as the number of school refusal cases I see continue to rise. I will recommend this book to every parent that I work with, school system I interact with, and mental health professional. Our children deserve better...they deserve to be healthy while also being educated.

—Denisha Johnson Hamilton, LCSW, CCATP | Outpatient Mental Health Therapist

As a parent and mental health advocate, reading *Improving School Mental Health* was a breath of fresh air and gave me a glimmer of hope for our school systems and families. In this book, Dr. Cam and Charle acknowledge and address real problems with realistic solutions and reasoning. Every educator, parent, and student will benefit and thrive from the wisdom and knowledge that spill from these pages.

—Jamie Edelbrock | Author and Mental Health Advocate

Schools during the Covid-19 pandemic became separated and isolated. Teachers and students have loudly worn their hurt post-Covid as mental health issues and burnout became the norm. Something must change and this system is a great start. Mental Health awareness has to be proactive in nature and it comes from having the proper tools and vision to thrive. This system helps not only students, but also teachers, administrators, and even parents as we move forward. It helps foster lost relationships and build a strong foundation of support to help all involved.

—Ryan D. Pelkey, M.Ed. | Middle School Health and PE Teacher/ Administrator/Athletic Director

We know that children spend a significant portion of their childhood in the classroom, but why haven't we found a proven strategy to increase mental health in the school environment? I believe that the framework presented in *Improving School Mental Health* is the answer for parents and educators alike. As I have seen the overlap between school environments and the digital environment, I am thrilled that the Thriving School Community solution will also have positive effects on children in the digital environment. Improved school mental health is unquestionably a boon both in the classroom and online.

—Dr. Elizabeth Milovidov | Creator, digitalparentingcoach.com

Improving School Mental Health: The Thriving School Community Solution, by Charle Peck and Dr. Cameron Caswell, is the guide that teachers and school communities have desperately needed for years! This is more than just a theory. It is a framework that applies theory to practice using real-world examples to explain how students, parents, caregivers, teachers, counselors, and administrators must work together in order to establish safe and brave learning spaces where children flourish.

—Antonietta McGoey | Science Educator at LaGuardia High School of Music & Art, and Performing Arts, Chief Diversity Officer at uThinkIndigo

A simple, pragmatic approach like N. A. C. is part of the solution for students, parents, and educators. Dr. Cam Caswell and Charle Peck are right that better solutions were needed long before the current crisis. I navigated the mental health issues daily with students for twenty years on the front lines as a school counselor. I believe they have a powerful long-term proactive answer: the Thriving School Community.

—Donovan Dreyer | School Counselor

As a veteran educator, I have read a plethora of books on curriculum, providing instruction, and incorporating standards into the teaching practice, which are important aspects of education but do not address the inner landscape that embodies mental health. What I love about the book, *Improving School Mental Health: The Thriving School Community Solution* is how the 9 pillars in the framework presented by Peck and Caswell facilitate your ability to engage in deep reflection within and authentic ownership of your own behaviors. As they guide you through their approach, you learn to fortify your intrapersonal skills, and their framework leads you to enhance your interpersonal skills. Although this book is geared towards educators, the practical wisdom in these methods is applicable for anyone who wants to move towards self-actualization, which is the ultimate fulfillment of your potential. This is a must read for preservice and seasoned practitioners in the education system as well as those individuals who seek to evolve their consciousness.

—Traci Nicole Smith, PhD | Conscious-Driven Living Coach, Educator, Parent Advocate, and Writer

Finally! An educational framework that not only acknowledges that the mental health of educators is essential to the mental health of our students but addresses it as part of the solution. As I read *Improving School Mental Health: The Thriving School Community Solution*, I found myself nodding my head, saying "Yes" out loud, and feeling validated as an educator. Charlie Peck and Dr. Cameron Caswell present nine essential skills and many practical tools to empower teachers, students, and parents that can be used every day to help us all improve our mental health and thrive. The TSC movement is what we all need right now!

—Terri McDaid | 6th Grade Teacher

Improving School Mental Health is well-written and highlights the nuance of pediatric mental health. The authors emphasize the importance of understanding youth behaviors and enhancing a child's well-being. This book is unique because it offers valuable tools to interact with youth and will be a great resource to improve youth mental health in our school system. I strongly recommend it!

—Vivekananda Rachamallu MD | A diplomate of the American Board of Psychiatry and Neurology (ABPN)

Now more than ever, teachers and school leaders need to increase their proficiency in identifying and responding to the mental health challenges of our children. Charle and Dr. Cam have written a book that is clear, refreshing, inspiring, and sorely needed. It's well organized, and the frameworks are empowering. I highly recommend it to teachers and school leaders alike!

—Moshe Fried | LCSW, School Social Worker, Co-Founder, ClasStars

The Thriving School Community is brilliant! It is a clear and consistent plan that addresses the mental health crisis of our teens. All the while, providing a framework for ALL stakeholders: students, educators, and parents. Looking at our current system of "triaging" mental health in education and the obvious fallout from it, TSC is a proactive system to empower teachers, students, and parents using thoughtful evidence-based skills that ingeniously work together, finally. This is a "must read" for all educators. TSC is a positive and proactive tool in a currently reactive environment to truly make lasting positive change in the mental health crisis we all witness in our schools.

—Nicole Terryberry | High School Teacher

Why is mental wellness continuing to decrease in my students? How can I better connect to support them, even with everything else my profession demands? How can supporting my students' mental well-being help their achievement in the classroom? After fifteen years as an educator in high school classrooms, these questions are ones I continue to struggle with. Charle Peck and Dr. Cameron Caswell combine years of frontline experience working with teens and research-based information to create a unique and inspiring action-based approach that provides strategies that can be immediately implemented in a classroom. *Improving School Mental Health* is a must read for any educator wishing to better support their students.

—Kate Lennox | High School Department Lead

Improving School Mental Health: The Thriving School Community Solution is a must-read guide for educators, parents, and mental health clinicians who want to help children become their best possible selves. This book provides a comprehensive yet simple approach to fostering healthy relationships with children, in a supportive and nurturing way, ultimately changing one's perspective on how to view and tackle the mental health crisis facing children today. Seems like something we should have been doing all along.

—Stacy M. Meyers, LPCC, NCC

Charle and Cameron inspire action and urgency to help our students thrive in a difficult world. *Improving School Mental Health: Thriving School Community Solution* effectively guides independent and collaborative reflection, discussion, and decision-making. Frameworks, quotations, and stories add context to guide conversations about mental health to enhance responsiveness, empathy, reflection, listening, and communication.

—Dr. Erik Youngman | Assistant Superintendent of Teaching and Learning in Libertyville, Illinois

Improving School Mental Health outlines critical ways we can all impact youth in our communities, offering a life raft to school communities struggling in rocky waters. By equipping caring adults in school communities to positively influence youth, the community as a whole becomes more flexible in our ability to support youth and better prepare educators to meet their academic needs. By addressing well-meaning, but often damaging, practices and replacing with evidence-based solutions we empower both our schools and larger community to support the mental health needs of our youth.

—Amy Weber Hall | PhD, LPCA, CHES Adolescent Therapist

I highly recommend *Improving School Mental Health: The Thriving School Community Solution* by Charle Peck and Cameron Caswell. Charle has spoken to our pre-service education students before and has shared proven strategies for tackling mental health issues in schools. This book encompasses those ideas and is an excellent resource for educators who want to improve the mental health of students and faculty in schools.

—Ryan Alverson, Ph.D. | Associate Professor, College of Education

Thank you to Charle Peck and Dr. Cameron Caswell for sharing so much great information in this book! Teachers are asked more and more to help with their students' mental health and this book gives our future and current teachers skills to sneak mental health into their lessons and also gives them strategies to teach their students to help them develop skills to empower themselves.

—Joetta Browning | Director of Experimental Education and
   Clinical Placements

Charle and Dr. Cam exemplified the importance of owning our feelings while we make decisions. Sitting through the discomfort is imperative when problem-solving through an issue. Without this step, a solution may become a bandaid fix and not a system change. Readers will find the book, Improving School Mental Health, both helpful and enjoyable to read. I wish the title was, *Why didn't anyone tell me this before? A solution to improving School Mental Health*."

—Mina Jo Blazy, Phd. | Director of Research, Learning and Data

Mental health is a topic that should be on the lips and minds of us all. Peck and Caswell do an impeccable job of providing the reader with information and actionable steps to be used right away. This is one of those books that will change lives."

—Todd Nesloney | Director of Culture and Strategic Leadership

Improving School Mental Health

Table of Contents

Introduction

"Every great dream begins with a dreamer. Always remember, you have within you the strength, the patience, and the passion to reach for the stars to change the world."

–Harriet Tubman

There is a mental health crisis within the education system. School personnel are disenfranchised and burned out. Students are struggling and stressed out. Parents are discouraged and checked out.

The pandemic may have exacerbated these problems, but it certainly didn't cause them. These issues have plagued our school system for decades. The pandemic shook the system and revealed the flaws and vulnerabilities that already existed within our current mental health solutions. Schools have been trying to address this ubiquitous problem for decades, but the mental health of students, educators, and parents alike remain a major concern.

The good news is local, state, and federal governments are prioritizing spending to build up mental health support. This has created a huge window of opportunity to make a cultural shift in our school communities—right now. We can either continue to spend our time, energy, and resources on more of what we've been doing for the past thirty years (without the impact we had hoped for)[1] OR we can do something different.

We believe it's time to do something different.

Our Stories

We both saw a flawed school system from different perspectives: Charle, as a seasoned teacher-turned-therapist and Dr. Cam as an adolescent psychologist.

Charle's Story

I always knew I wanted to help teens navigate the challenges the world threw at them. They were sorely misunderstood—as I remembered from my own youth—and I believed there was much more to learn about this confusing, yet, fascinating, stage of life. As a high school teacher for eighteen years, I had the great benefit of educating teens about mental health, human development, and emerging brain science which afforded me years of learning and observation. I used this time to deeply understand adolescents and their school experience while studying the system and paying close attention to its strengths—as well as its glaring flaws. On a mission to spark mental health change on a massive scale, I took a risk and stepped out of teaching. I earned my Master of Social Work (MSW) and became a therapist to learn more about the dynamics of relationships, gaining a clinical lens to help identify deep-rooted personal, social, and structural issues that plague our youth along the way. After several years in this experiential role, I realized that any change must happen first with the adults in our kids' lives. Since children and teens split much of their time between home

---

[1] APA, 2009

and school, I assert that we must invest in the mental health of school staff and caregivers.

Dr. Cam's Story

I'd been working with teens and tweens and their families as a family coach. In my practice, I was getting an influx of pleas for help from parents worried about their children's lack of motivation and resistance to school, increasing anxiety, low self-esteem, and challenging attitude. When I talked to their children, I heard the same thing over and over again: school is boring, their educators hate them, their parents only care about their grades, not who they were. They would say to me, "I can't do anything right. Why even bother? I give up." If this many children and families were having the same problems and worries, it seemed more logical that the issue wasn't with them, but with the system. I love working with families, but the number of people in need far outnumber the people available to help them. I knew that if I was going to make a real difference, I had to help whole communities rather than individuals. When I crossed paths with Charle through our podcasts, we immediately realized how well our visions aligned.

The Story of Us

After years of working with adolescents and families, we were each seeing problems that emerged from the school environment. Compelled to help families navigate conflict, Dr. Cam started a podcast, *Parenting Teens with Dr. Cam,* and designed a successful program supporting teens and their parents. Charle took a similar approach and started a podcast called *Advancing Humanity* and designed workshops for educators and school staff. Ultimately, we were each trying to strengthen these two crucial systems (schools and families) so kids could thrive within them.

We first asked each other to be guests on one another's podcast, and the connection was apparent. We both had the same passion for kids and families and concluded that school is where youth spend much of their time[2] and where many of our kids' problems both manifest and fester. Yet, we kept throwing kids back into toxic environments and expecting them to succeed. It felt like madness; we knew we had to do something BIG if we were going to make a significant impact in the work we aimed to do. We believed schools have a responsibility to strengthen their relationship with parents and vice versa, so all adults could work together to support kids. After hours of discussion, we came up with a plan to work our magic. And so was born: Thriving School Community (TSC).

The Story of TSC

For the past two years we've debated, shared our experiences, talked with educators, students, and parents, and tested our concepts and strategies through our private practices to determine what really works. We refined and simplified until we landed on a sustainable plan to improve student behaviors, well-being, and academic outcomes leveraging the power of the school community. We then took our ideas on the road, teaching them to educators and parents across the United States. The response has been overwhelming! Educators tell us they usually dread professional development, but our approach helped them feel "energized" and "better equipped." Parents told us they believe if they had learned our solutions earlier it would have saved them a lot of heartache and frustration. Almost everyone told us they wanted to learn more. Many pleaded for us to put what we teach into a book. And so we did.

---

[2] U.S. Department of Health and Human Services Centers for Disease Control and Prevention (2022)

This book provides the framework for the TSC solution to the student mental health crisis, offering practical tools and strategies for educators to foster well-being for themselves and their students today.

The Dilemma

In 2021, the American Academy of Pediatrics declared child and adolescent mental health a national emergency.[3] During the COVID-19 pandemic, depression, anxiety, self-harm, and suicidality skyrocketed. Although isolation, fear, and uncertainty exacerbated these mental health concerns, this crisis has been a serious problem for decades. The pandemic merely exposed how vulnerable our state of mental health already was, showing we didn't have a strong enough foundation to withstand it.

Forty percent of students sitting in your building report having persistent feelings of sadness or hopelessness.[4] 40%! Youth depressive and anxiety symptoms doubled during the pandemic though an astounding 88% of schools are not confident they can support their students' mental health. So kids are spending a large portion of their time thinking about, stressing over, and going to school, but the people, the practices, and the processes within this system remain ill-equipped to respond to their needs. The system is failing them.

School districts collect an ample amount of data, so we know where the gaps are. However, many don't have the time, bandwidth, or expertise to figure out what to do with all the data.

The Blame Game

We're trying to fix mental health by teaching students skills to become more resilient. The problem is, we're thinking about it wrong.

---

[3] American Academy of Child and Adolescent Psychiatry (2022)
[4] The U.S. Surgeon General's Advisory (2021)

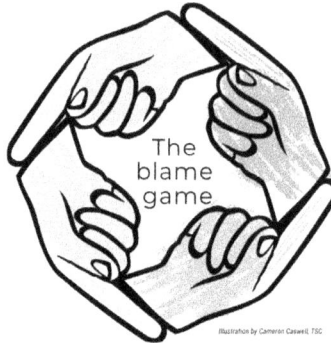

Illustration by Cameron Caswell, TSC

We're trying to solve the problem by teaching our students social skills and emotional regulation. However, no matter how many classes, lectures, and programs we deliver, the second we throw them back into an environment with burned out educators and stressed out parents, they're going to revert back to the same discouraging behavior. Out of frustration in dealing with the same patterns, we resort to blame:

+ If students would just behave
+ If parents would be more engaged
+ If educators could be more engaging
+ If administrators were more supportive
+ If funding was more accessible.

When we get stuck in the blame game, we contribute to a fractured school mental health system rather than improving it.

Three Problems to Address

It's tough for kids to learn when they're struggling with mental health, disengaged, or avoiding school altogether. To facilitate real change, we must address the following problems:

Problem 1: We're using piecemeal products that are not compatible in an attempt to improve student wellness. We waste time and money on solutions that check the boxes but don't fit together well.

Think about it like this: You go to get dressed and realize you have a lot of pants and plenty of shirts hanging in your closet. You've also got shoes, jackets, and varied accessories. Yet, nothing matches, and you don't have a complete outfit to wear. Now think of products you've purchased for your school to improve student mental health. Like your wardrobe, you've got a lot to choose from, but chances are they don't all work together to deliver a complete solution.

Problem 2: Educators are overburdened and unequipped to respond to the effects of the youth mental health crisis. Add to that the fact that their own mental health is suffering.

Think about it like this: You're getting ready to send your child on a flight across the Atlantic. As your child boards the plane, the flight attendant says, "Don't worry, we've got your kid for the duration of the trip. Trust us, we're trained in all the emergency procedures." You feel a sense of relief, but then unease. You say, "O.K., but what happens if my child starts to panic when there's turbulence?" The flight attendant responds, "Well, we're not trained to handle that, but if there is a major problem, we've got it covered." You're glad there's a plan in place for big emergencies, but those rarely happen.

We're sending our children on these regular "flights" who need varied supports. We want them to feel secure so they can enjoy the ride. A few "crew members" are highly trained to keep them safe if there is a fire or a lockdown; however, they don't know how to effectively respond to our kids' needs when it gets bumpy. And if they're already stressed out, how are they going to figure it out in the middle of a crisis?

Problem 3: We get forced into a reactive state of triage trying to stop as many youth from drowning as we can.

Think about it like this: Imagine you're strolling along a riverbank and see a bunch of kids drifting along struggling to stay afloat. Some are silently treading water while others are crying out for help. Many are clearly drowning. You immediately reach for kids to pull them out to safety but don't even know where to begin. As more and more keep coming, you realize there's no way to get to them all. You've never felt so helpless. Our schools are backlogged with children who are essentially drowning in mental health issues. As long as we continue reacting to the problems rather than preventing them, they're going to continue flooding our system.

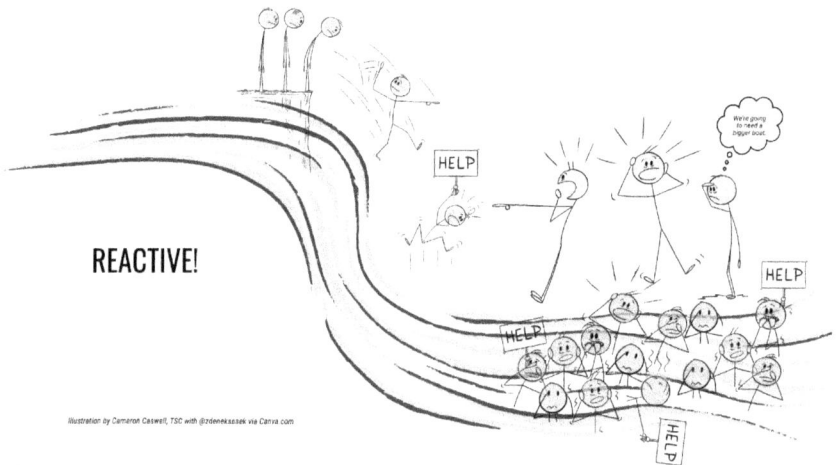

REACTIVE!

Illustration by Cameron Caswell, TSC with @zdenekasasek via Canva.com

PART I

~

The TSC Solution

What is the Thriving School Community?

The Thriving School Community (TSC) is a comprehensive, yet simpler approach to effectively restore, strengthen, and sustain the mental health of staff and students without adding MORE to do. The TSC mission is to:

+ Energize Educators
+ Empower Students
+ Engage Parents

The goal of this program is to ignite a systemic mental health transformation by fostering positive, cooperative partnerships among educators, parents, and students. Ultimately, TSC creates an immersive experience that fosters well-being at school and at home.

The TSC Framework

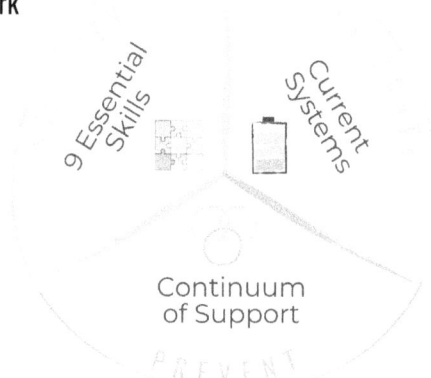

The TSC Framework is designed to simplify the solution, integrate current systems, and prevent further problems from occurring.

The TSC Framework

9 Essential Skills

Current Systems

Continuum of Support

PREVENT

Illustration by Cameron Caswell, TSC

1. SIMPLIFY: Focus on nine evidence-based skills. These fit together like puzzle pieces to form a complete solution rather than using piecemeal products that aren't compatible. Instead of investing more in complex programs and major overhauls, focus on teaching and reinforcing these nine skills. Together, these nine skills build a sturdy foundation for well-being.

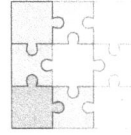

   They are grouped into three skill sets:

   Auto Skills (SELF)

   Allo Skills (OTHER)

   Ambi Skills (TOGETHER)

   These skills:

   + are easy to understand and implement with practical tools and strategies so they'll be readily utilized.
   + assess behaviors as symptoms of an underlying problem rather than the problem itself.
   + reflect the essence of how we understand ourselves, relate to others, and work together.

2. INTEGRATE: Power up your current systems. You already have amazing educators in place. This framework helps them maintain their own mental health and wellness and reminds them of their value. They will feel supported and equipped to handle their busy workload in addition to student mental health issues confidently. Since the skills are infused into daily practice, wellness seamlessly flows into everyday life. Finally, with clear guidance on what to do when common mental health issues arise, it removes the guesswork. We do this by powering up your:

+ people
+ practices
+ protocols

By taking these steps, it alleviates strain on the entire system.

3. PREVENT: Establish a continuum of support. We're bridging the gap among key pillars of the school community to prevent mental health issues from occurring or burgeoning. These pillars are:
   + educators
   + students
   + parents/caregivers

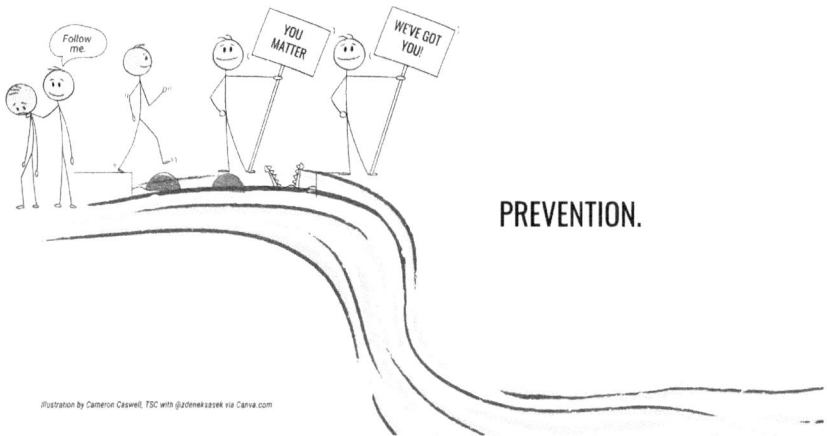

PREVENTION.

Illustration by Cameron Caswell, TSC with @deneksasek via Canva.com

Since all are of equal value, all are equipped with the nine essential skills. When we create an immersive experience with everyone practicing, modeling, and building proficiency, we propagate a supportive culture that can withstand changing leadership and initiatives.

CHAPTER 1

Focus on Nine Essential Skills

"Give a person an idea, and you can enrich their day.
Teach a person how to learn, and they can enrich their entire life."

–Jim Kwik, Limitless

Sam is a sophomore student who attends a large, well-funded high school. There are 9 school counselors, a social worker, and a psychologist all onsite. There is an abundance of leadership, character development, and peer support programs, and recently, a spirited school-wide pep rally was held to kick off their "Depression Awareness" campaign. Sam sees an external therapist to help him manage anxiety and is standing by his locker one morning when he feels a panic attack coming on.

Dr. Diaz, Sam's therapist, is in the middle of a meeting and hears her phone buzz. It's a text from Sam:

Sam: "I'm having an anxiety attack."

Dr. Diaz: "Where are you?"

Sam: "School"

Dr. Diaz is worried. She doesn't want Sam to be alone.

Dr. Diaz: "Is there someone you can talk to at school? A counselor?"

Sam: "Not really. My old counselor left, and I don't know the new one."

Dr. Diaz: "How about one of your teachers?"

Sam: "I can't. They barely even know me."

Sam is surrounded by caring adults and plenty of mental health supports, yet feels completely alone.

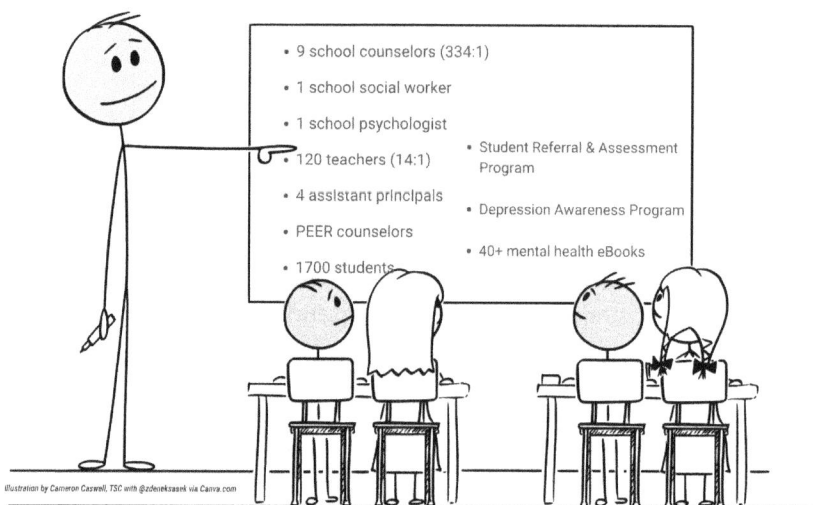

Illustration by Cameron Caswell, TSC with @zdeneksasek via Canva.com

- 9 school counselors (334:1)
- 1 school social worker
- 1 school psychologist
- 120 teachers (14:1)
- 4 assistant principals
- PEER counselors
- 1700 students
- Student Referral & Assessment Program
- Depression Awareness Program
- 40+ mental health eBooks

Despite all the mental health resources at this school (see above image), Sam still struggled in isolation and, tragically, attempted suicide later that day. When the products, services, and supports do not work as a cohesive, thriving system, kids like Sam get left behind.

Putting the Pieces Together

The nine skills fit together like a cohesive puzzle. They are all we need to make the necessary shifts in youth mental health, laying the foundation for meaningful connections with kids. Because we build trusting relationships, we become more approachable and cultivate a safe learning environment. This also encourages students to advocate for themselves, asking for what they need. If Sam felt secure in his school environment, he may have reached out for help there.

These nine skills are rooted in behavioral health which helps us form a better narrative about student behavior. Behavior is a symptom, not the problem itself. Even when we don't know any details about underlying issues, we at least acknowledge there is more going on than what we're seeing so we can appropriately respond.

When we have the tools, we serve as good informants for mental health experts who are trained to consider contributing factors to the child's problem. For Sam, we may have noticed shifts in work, performance, or mood, for example, and could have better described our observations. Sometimes we can reconcile the underlying issue with the child to meet a need more readily on our own. Regardless, when we are connected and provide security for students, they don't slip through the cracks.

With this complete, yet simple, approach, the system functions as an interconnected network adding protective factors for children in our schools. Because it's easy to implement and provides practical tools and strategies, it brings fractured systems together quickly and has both immediate and long-term impact. Imagine the result for Sam if all of those resources were in place like this.

The TSC framework has the power to kickstart significant change in your school mental health system. Ready for it? Let's get started.

The Nine Essential Skills

The Auto, Allo, and Ambi skills are grouped so that all the important aspects of a thriving system are covered:

- *Auto skills* help us understand *ourselves*.
- *Allo skills* help us relate to *others*.
- *Ambi skills* help us work *together*.

Each contain three specific skills showing how to:

- *protect* our sense of self, others, and our relationships.
- *connect* to ourselves, to others, and together.
- *resolve* issues within ourselves, with others, and together.

Each of these individual skills has a designated chapter within this book so you can learn when to use it, why to use it, and how to use it.

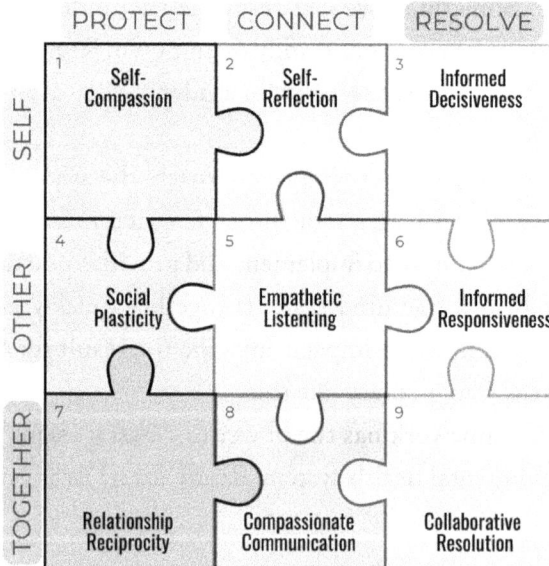

	PROTECT	CONNECT	RESOLVE
SELF	1 Self-Compassion	2 Self-Reflection	3 Informed Decisiveness
OTHER	4 Social Plasticity	5 Empathetic Listening	6 Informed Responsiveness
TOGETHER	7 Relationship Reciprocity	8 Compassionate Communication	9 Collaborative Resolution

Illustration by Cameron Caswell, TSC

To demonstrate how these skills teach you to assess behavior and interpret it in a meaningful way, let's consider an incident shared with us by a teacher we worked with, who we'll call Ms. Bandura:

> When her freshman student, Anya, disrupted her science lab by leaving the room (without permission), Ms. Bandura was annoyed. She attempted to approach Anya after class, though she quickly slipped out when the bell rang. Ms. Bandura was called to the office soon after and told by the principal to "ignore it" when Anya leaves the room without explanation. Confused but compliant in the following weeks, Ms. Bandura built up frustration towards Anya each time she left. Anya became distant and often gave Ms. Bandura "attitude" during their interactions. Wanting to make amends, Ms. Bandura sought her out after school one day but sadly learned that Anya had passed away. Anya had a terminal illness that warranted frequent bathroom breaks. She was embarrassed about this and wanted to keep her illness confidential so she could be treated "like a normal kid." Ms. Bandura was guilt-ridden, heartbroken, and left with overwhelming thoughts of "if I only knew..."

We believe Ms. Bandura didn't need to know the specifics of Anya's illness to have been a good support for her. Children sit in our classrooms with varying ailments and adversity we will never know about. If we are proficient in the nine essential skills, we can still make connections and provide a safe, inclusive learning space for them. Ms. Bandura could have enhanced her experience with more compassion and avoided the tremendous guilt she carried after Anya passed. She could have adjusted her mindset and had practical tools to support her instead. She would have established a rapport and connection with Anya regardless of her "behaviors" and feel less stressed. Simply,

Ms. Bandura would have the capacity to think critically about Anya's behavior altogether.

Striving for Proficiency, Not Perfection

Educators who are equipped with these nine skills cope well with stress and effectively teach students through challenges, even when they're still working on building proficiency. They build capacity to manage their emotions and have peaceful exchanges with others so they can focus on the work they love. They competently establish connected classrooms and secure environments that become safe havens for kids. It's evident that educators want to support their students' mental health, and in most cases are already doing the best they can; they just want tools to respond *better*. They care, and they want students feeling confident and willing (maybe even excited?!) to learn.

The Biggest Takeaways

1. Behavior is a symptom of the problem, not the problem itself.
2. We must create deeper connections with students to foster more secure learning environments.
3. The nine skills fit together like a cohesive puzzle. By keeping the program simple and easy to implement, immediate change can begin today.

CHAPTER 2

~

Power Up Your
Current Systems

"After persevering through the hardest school years in memory, America's educators are exhausted and increasingly burned out… This crisis is preventing educators from giving their students the one-on-one attention they need….and is preventing students from getting the mental health supports needed."

–NEA (2022)

The bell is about to ring any minute now, and Mr. Brown scrambles to get his notes ready before his next class starts. He looks up to see Ryan, one of his 6th grade students, standing in front of him. Ryan is usually very calm and collected, but Mr. Brown notices something is off. Ryan says, "Can I talk to you?" Although Mr. Brown definitely doesn't have the time, he can see Ryan is on the verge of tears, and there's no way he can say no. His student clearly needs help right now, but thirty other students are filing in. Mr. Brown encourages Ryan to talk to the school social worker after school. Ryan hesitates, "But you're the only one I trust." Mr. Brown feels powerless.

This scenario with Ryan is common. Children often build trusting relationships with educators, but it becomes overwhelming to be their regular confidant when we're busy and don't have the know-how to respond. We have compassion for them, and we know that when kids function well, they behave better and are more productive, so meaningful learning takes place[2]. This makes our jobs much easier and reduces overwhelm for both of us.

Remember Sam, the student with a school full of mental health resources from Ch. 1? If the system was more interconnected, Sam may have felt more comfortable approaching school staff for help. When equipped with the nine essential skills, the system works more efficiently and is inviting to students like Sam.

But what if you've already invested in products to get your mental health system functioning well? Do you just toss them aside to make room for a big overhaul? Not at all. The TSC framework utilizes what's working well in your building. The nine skills integrate into your current system to power up what you already have in place including your:

+ people.
+ practices.
+ protocols.

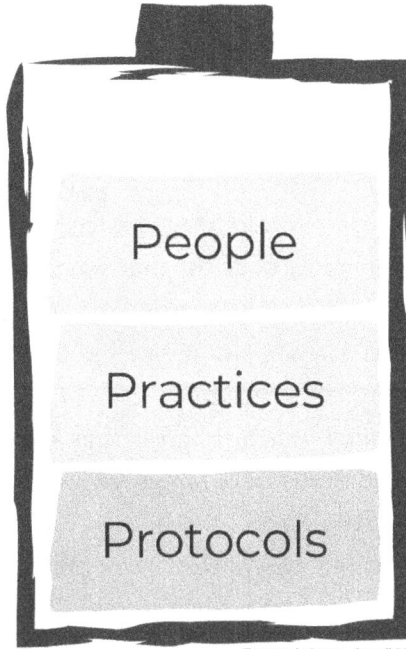

Illustration by Cameron Caswell, TSC

Power Up Your People

The success of any school mental health program is contingent upon the ability of staff to implement it. Two barriers to this are burnout and being unequipped to deliver it effectively.

Ninety percent of National Education Association (NEA) members reported that burnout is a critical issue plaguing our education system.[5] The cycle starts with good intentions, but after an educator has to deal with student misbehavior over and over, they get frustrated and eventually give up.

---

[5] Walker - National Education Association (NEA) 2022

Mr. Kim, is a teacher who spends hours planning fun, engaging lessons for his senior students. Ten minutes into his introduction of the Civil War, a few students act out and disrupt the lesson flow. He spends the next ten minutes attempting to get a small group of students to stop interrupting, but they persist. Now other students lose interest. Mr. Kim feels disdain towards the "troublemakers" because of all the time wasted. He is drained and disheartened. Again. He has to rethink and reorganize his lessons using up his next sacred planning period. As a result, he has to put off the phone call he was going to make to Talia's foster mom to let her know how much progress she's made this past week. That kid deserved a celebratory message, and Mr. Kim's intention was there, but he couldn't follow through. At the next staff meeting, educators, including Mr. Kim, were called out for neglecting to make positive calls home. Mr. Kim rolls his eyes and wonders, "What am I doing here? This isn't what I signed up for."

How can educators support kids when they feel burned out themselves? They can't. Or won't. And they are leaving the profession in droves.

Here is what the N.E.A. proposed to handle teacher burnout (see chart):

Proposed Solutions for Burnout

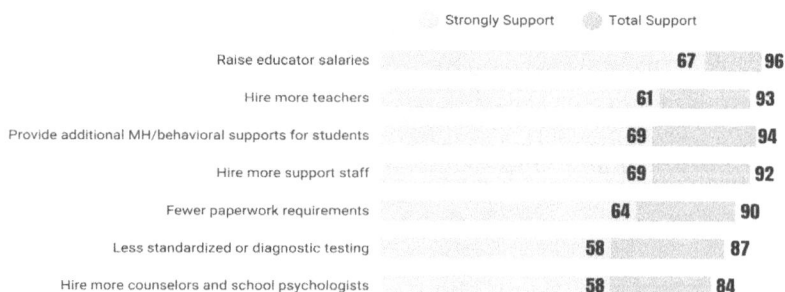

	Strongly Support	Total Support
Raise educator salaries	67	96
Hire more teachers	61	93
Provide additional MH/behavioral supports for students	69	94
Hire more support staff	69	92
Fewer paperwork requirements	64	90
Less standardized or diagnostic testing	58	87
Hire more counselors and school psychologists	58	84

NEA. Solutions to the Educator Shortage Crisis (2022)

What do most of these have in common? They have us doing MORE.

MORE pay.

MORE staff.

MORE resources.

MORE for everyone to do.

For decades, we've been trying to solve the problem by throwing more at it, yet mental health continues to decline.[6]

We've had 20 years of adding more than double the amount of mental health reinforcements, but still, we have high rates of anxiety, suicide, and depression among youth.[7]

We need to stop throwing more at educators adding to their to-do list, and instead, give them what they've been asking for: reduce their level of feeling overwhelmed. The TSC framework does this by equipping educators with practical tools to first manage their own wellness and then to help students navigate theirs.

Ninety-three percent of educators say they are ill-equipped to handle student mental health issues.[8] They aren't trying to be their students' therapists, nor are we asking them to. However, they are the first line of defense, so when they lack skills or knowledge to aptly respond or set healthy limits, it can be draining.

Let's go back to Ryan, the student who asked Mr. Brown for help at the beginning of this chapter. If Mr. Brown had proficiency in the Allo skills when Ryan approached him, he could use a temporary intervention to keep Ryan in the classroom until he could get help. Ryan's learning wouldn't be disrupted, and Mr. Brown wouldn't feel so powerless.

---

[6] American Psychological Association (2022)

[7] American Psychological Association (2022)

[8] American Psychiatric Association Public Opinion Poll (2021)

Teachers say...

93%

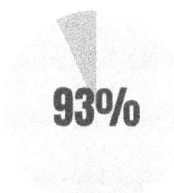

are concerned about
students' mental
well-being, but feel
ill-prepared to respond.

American Psychiatric Association Public Opinion Poll (2021)

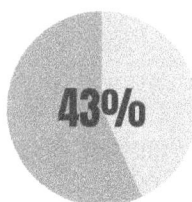

43%

the stress and
disappointments of
teaching **aren't worth it.**

State of the U.S. Teacher Survey (2021)

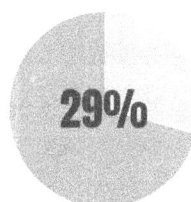

29%

they **don't get enough
support** from their
district or school

State of the U.S. Teacher Survey (2021)

Whether it's a part of their job description or not, educators want to help. We are packed full of expert, loving, compassionate people who show up for students every day, so let's focus on better equipping those rockstar educators who are already in your building.

"...as the unthinkable toll of the shooting came into focus, some parents texted the teacher: "Thank you for keeping my baby safe."

"But it's not just their baby," the teacher said, sobbing on her front porch. "That's my baby, too. They are not my students. They are my children." From a teacher at the Uvalde school Hixenbaugh (2022).

Power Up Your Practices

If you're teaching mental health as a separate class or task (e.g., Advisory, Wellness Wednesdays, targeted leadership or character programs, video series, etc.), and it's resolving your mental health issues, great, keep doing that! You don't need to change what's working well. If your staff is struggling to keep up with it all, and mental health is still an issue, however, it may be time to integrate something simpler into your current programming. Teaching wellness strategies and topics as a separate class or activity adds to the workload and creates inconsistency. Although there is extraordinary value in multilayered programs, they create a heavy load for educators and staff. These can also create a barrier with parents if there is miscommunication or if they are uninvolved. The TSC framework proposes to seamlessly infuse wellness into everyday practice instead. That way, we make big gains with less to do. Additionally, educators manage their own wellness all day long while cultivating a healthy, vibrant learning space for students. The nine skills become reflexive practice and student mental health improves with less strain on the system.

If you're worried about parent buy-in, National Alliance on Mental Illness (NAMI) found that parents are deeply concerned about their children's wellness, too, and strongly support having it addressed within our school system. Eighty-nine percent said their child's mental health matters more than their academic achievement, and 87% say mental health education should be taught in schools.[9] BUT…we don't want educators and staff feeling like they have to learn, plan, and deliver a whole new curriculum.

Power Up Your Protocols

After equipping educators and teaching them how to infuse the nine skills into daily practice, we need to reduce even more pressure by refining your protocols, for example, your student referral process. This takes the guesswork out of what to do when common mental health issues and emergencies occur.

Educators are only referring their students to mental health professionals 19% of the time while over half of them report handling

---

[9] National Alliance on Mental Illness (NAMI), 2021

student issues themselves.[10] No wonder they're feeling burnout—it's a heavy load to carry. How do we improve this situation so kids can get the expert help they need, and teachers feel less strain? Let's first look at why educators aren't doing this. Here's what they're telling us:

+ There is no system in place that is easy and immediate.
+ There is a lack of communication back to the teacher when they do refer students, so they aren't confident it's working.
+ There aren't enough mental health professionals to manage the overwhelming numbers, so they don't trust it will help. Even in the well-funded school Sam attended from Chapter 1, the caseloads were still exceedingly high, so kids connected more with their teachers, not the skilled counselors.

Consider your referral process (if you have one).

+ Is it used consistently? If so, by whom? If not, why not?
+ Is feedback provided to the person who made the referral?
+ Does an incident report need to be filled out?
+ Does a Child Protective Services report need to be completed? If so, who will do that?
+ Does the child's guardian need to be contacted? If so, who will make that call?
+ Which protective factors will be added when the child returns to the classroom?

These are just a few questions to consider when refining a protocol like this. It's important to identify gaps and get feedback from staff, students, and parents to ensure it's functioning the way it's intended to. You may have to ask educators what they need to do their jobs better,

---

[10] National Survey by the University of South Carolina, George Mason University, Loyola University Chicago + the University of Missouri (2020)

for example, and try to help them get that. You already have loads of data from incredible products you've invested in; now it's time to put these data to good use.

We know how to escape a building when there is a fire, but does everyone in your building know how to respond to a mental health crisis? If Mr. Brown knew the protocol to quickly refer Ryan, he could free up mental energy to teach his class. Ryan would also have a team of resources to look forward to. When your mental health protocols are refined (or added), based on identified needs, an integrated network of support emerges. In a thriving school community, we have a seamless exchange of information affording less room to err with clearly defined procedures to protect everyone involved.

The Biggest Takeaways

1. Since educators are regular confidants, equipping them with tools to respond effectively to students will reduce stress and feelings of being overwhelmed.
2. When educators infuse the nine essential skills into daily practice, they consistently manage their own wellness and establish a healthy learning environment for students.
3. You don't need major overhauls to improve student mental health; you can power up what you already have in place to start building an integrated network of support.

CHAPTER 3

⌒

Establish a Continuum of Support

"Alone we can do so little; Together we can do so much."

–Helen Keller

The final component of the TSC framework is to establish a continuum of support by investing in ALL three pillars of the school community: educators, parents, and students. Addressing one without the others creates imbalance while having strength in all three creates homeostasis.

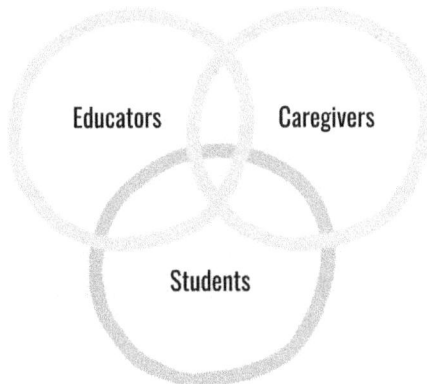

Educators   Caregivers

Students

Imagine you're driving late at night and get hit by an oncoming truck that swerved into your lane. You are ejected from your car and lay on the cold pavement. Someone calls 911, and EMTs show up. They immediately do an assessment and get to work stabilizing you. One of the EMTs talks calmly to reassure you while the other communicates their observations of any obvious injuries or signs of trauma to dispatch. Because doctors received these details before you arrive, they now have some indication of how to treat you, and, therefore, you get the help you need more swiftly. Meanwhile, your closest relative is en route to be at your side because staff followed protocol and reached out to them. You may have avoided catastrophic damage altogether, or at the very least, you weren't curled up alone on the side of the road suffering in silence.

Picture educators as first responders. They have tools to stabilize (or calm) a student who is struggling and can effectively gather information that will be helpful to mental health professionals. Students advocate for what they need, and parents contribute a historical background. All are great informants and integral parts of the team but don't require the clinical training professionals do. "Frontline" staff now feel competent,[11] parents feel less overwhelmed, and students get the care they need instead of feeling left behind.

---

[11] The educators we work with tell us that they are rarely asked to share their perspectives. Instead of consulting them as a valued resource, they are frequently excluded from the process. We know there are issues with confidentiality around mental health which needs to be honored, but there is still room for teacher input.

Prevention, Not Reaction

To prevent mental health issues from feverishly occurring, we link in parents and any adult who interacts with our kids. Adults model the skills and encourage kids to use them. Imagine all pillars practicing the nine skills within the culture building proficiency *together*. Like an immersive language experience, when the skills become habitual and reflexive, there is fluency. When we have an entire school community doing this, we witness the results of a thriving school community.

In turn, we prevent issues from getting bigger. Sometimes kids like Ryan, who approached his teacher for help in Chapter 2, resort to more explosive behaviors when they struggle, setting off a defensive reaction by adults. When we are unequipped, we typically lead with anger and frustration. Consequently, when everyone is equipped, we let student behavior tell us their story and respond effectively. Kids gain trust in adults and in the mental health system again. They now have somewhere accessible and reliable to turn to when they need help.

The Stress Spillover

Kids feel stress from both the school and home environment which impacts their state of wellbeing. Because a child's homelife influences their learning experience, even long-term,[12] it's in our schools' best interest to partner with parents. It is particularly important for students in vulnerable populations who are underserved and marginalized.[13]

Parents are often overwhelmed and struggle to effectively raise their kids and are provided limited guidance.[14] Kids act out when parenting

---

[12] Warner (2008)

[13] https://safesupportivelearning.ed.gov/sites/default/files/13-ImpSchMn-HlthSprtBtPrt-508_0.pdf

[14] https://www.zerotothree.org/resource/national-parent-survey-overview-and-key-insights/

skills are lacking. Those behaviors show up in our schools, compounding the problem. Before the pandemic, teaching was already identified as one of the most stressful occupations in the U.S.[15] Now, with the added stress of student misbehavior, educators are overloaded. When educators and parents both have a low ability to regulate themselves, student outcomes are negatively impacted.[16] When students have trouble at school, it leads to more stress at home;[17] hence, the cycle is perpetuated in both environments. This is what is known as stress spillover.[18]

When kids move back and forth between settings with deflated adults who lack the energy and competency to provide them with what they need, they lose faith in the systems that are supposed to support them. They eventually lose trust in all adults. They may even lose faith in humanity. They detach from everyone. They fall into an oblivion of isolation and don't feel like they matter. They run out of hope. So they attempt (or tragically complete) suicide, self-harm, commit crimes, engage in risky sexual behaviors, latch on to abusive partners, question their identity, lose their self-worth, punch, kick, scream. They're angry and frustrated. They feel alone. And they are alone.

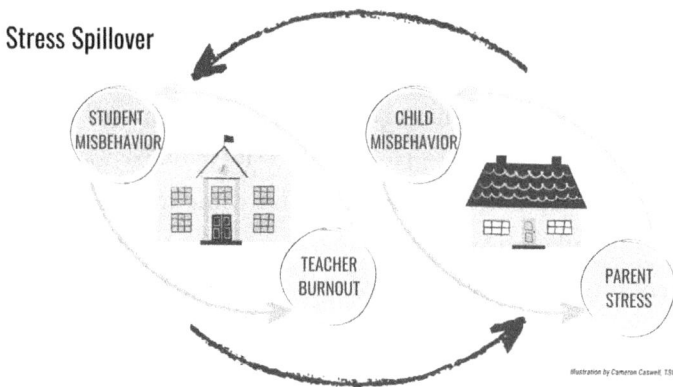

Stress Spillover

STUDENT MISBEHAVIOR

CHILD MISBEHAVIOR

TEACHER BURNOUT

PARENT STRESS

Illustration by Cameron Caswell, TSC

---

[15] Robert Wood Johnson Foundation (2017)

[16] Herman et al. (2018)

[17] Warner (2008)

[18] file:///C:/Users/charl/Downloads/fpsyg-13-909928.pdf

We are desperately trying to fix our kids' problems so they can function and find some joy in a culture burdened with depression, anxiety, PTSD, psychosis, and other debilitating issues resulting from childhood or complex trauma and other ailments. The problem is, we're trying to teach students to better manage *themselves* but then throw them right back into the same stressful environments that cause the issues in the first place. This leaves them little chance to thrive.

In Chapter 2, we demonstrated the importance of equipping educators, though we only help our kids when we equip parents too.

Creating a Sustainable Ecosystem

A recent study released by the National PTA evidenced that children are more resilient when parents partner with schools.[19] [20] Research repeatedly correlates family engagement with student achievement, so it would be a disservice not to include this strategy in mental health reform.[21] Current solutions may unintentionally leave parents out or have challenges with communication[22] so the TSC framework is structured with parents[23] in mind. Here's what we're currently hearing from educators with whom we work:

+ There is fear of being blamed for student behavior when reaching out to parents.

---

[19] https://safesupportivelearning.ed.gov/sites/default/files/13-ImpSchMn-HlthSprtBtPrt-508_0.pdf

[20] Dr. Ethier - PTA.org (2022)

[21] Weiss et al, 2010; Project Appleseed (2022). https://www.projectappleseed.org/barriers

[22] Baker et al. (2016) p. 171

[23] Including caregivers, guardians, custodial parents.

+ Educators feel pressure to handle student behaviors themselves. When they get to the point of involving parents, they feel like they've failed or worry they will appear incompetent.
+ Staff shy away from parents when trying to solve student behavior issues which contributes to their exhaustion.

Parents also feel disconnected. Though they appear to be working against schools, we've learned from parents that they are simply frustrated and feel excluded. Here's what we're hearing:

+ Poor communication makes parents perceive the school to be "less family-friendly." [24]
+ Parents need to feel a sense of belonging in the school community in order to become more involved. Otherwise, they avoid it altogether.
+ Parents express concern that they receive communication about their child's progress (or lack thereof) only after major problems occur. At this point, they're shocked, disappointed, and embarrassed, and they vent elsewhere.

Separating ourselves from each other won't help the mental health crisis. Our school climate functions as a result of the connect or disconnect between members of the school community, so coming together has to be a part of the solution. The relationship among staff is important, too. If you've ever worked in an environment with disenfranchised educators, you know that tension radiates throughout the entire building and can be felt by everyone, including outsiders.

When we create an ecosystem of support, kids feel connected and have what they need to thrive.[25] Disruptive behaviors (e. g., fighting,

---

[24] Baker et al. (2016) p. 170

[25] Cara McNulty, president of behavioral health and mental well-being at CVS Health.

attendance avoidance, and suspension rates) will decrease and more positive ones (e. g., an increase in credit completion and graduation rates) will arise.[26] When we learn about the whole child experience in both the school and family environment, we can provide reinforcements in both places.

Sharing the burden of raising healthy, well-functioning children in today's demanding world provides relief to all adults involved. By being proactive rather than reactive, we strengthen the entire system, and we add a layer of protection to prevent problems from occurring in the first place. Because we're building proficiency through an immersive cultural experience, the system is sustainable. This is how we establish a continuum of support.

Shifting Responsibility From a Few to Many

Imagine everyone being equipped with these nine skills to manage themselves, respond well to others, and work better together. It shifts the responsibility of student mental health from just a few professionals in the building to everyone. Your mental health staff has more time to dedicate to students with complex issues. Maladaptive behaviors lessen since there are more opportunities to be heard and expressive in a space of acceptance and kindness. Ultimately, we build a more peaceful, thriving school culture where the nine essential skills are normalized.[27]

The Biggest Takeaways

1. With all pillars working harmoniously together, we alleviate strain on the entire education system.
2. When we equip parents with the nine essential skills, we produce better learners.

---

[26] https://files.eric.ed.gov/fulltext/ED595733.pdf
[27] McCombs School of Business (2022)

3. When we are all trained to model and reinforce the same skills consistently, we make a transformational shift in both school and home culture.

PART II

~

The Nine Essential Skills

In this section we dive deeper into the nine behavioral health skills that are foundational to the TSC framework. These skills streamline complicated concepts to make it easier for us to:

1. Protect ourselves, others, and our relationships.
2. Connect with ourselves, with others, and within a relationship.
3. Resolve our own problems, issues with others, and challenges within a relationship.

An Overview of Auto Skills (Self/Me)

Auto skills are the foundation for self. They are core to understanding and managing our self-perceptions, choices, values, biases, and beliefs. They focus on meeting your own needs so you can show up energized for your staff and students. Auto skills also enable us to make decisions without feeling paralyzed by external pressures and take ownership and accountability for our choices and actions without shame. They tap into our own strengths and help us overcome challenges which build up a sense of agency, boost our self-confidence, and foster empathy and compassion for not only others, but also for ourselves. We all deserve to experience the peace this brings, and the people we care about will benefit from getting the best of us as an added bonus.

We've identified three Auto skills: Self-Compassion (Chapter 4), Self-Reflection (Chapter 5), and Informed Decisiveness (Chapter 6).

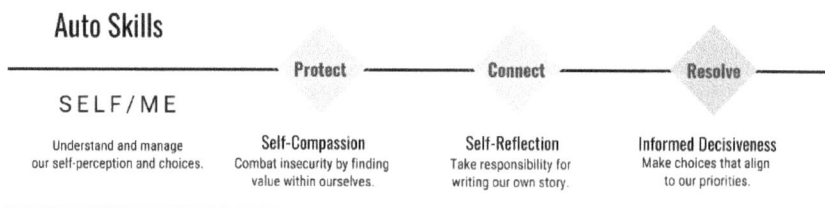

Auto Skills

	Protect	Connect	Resolve
SELF/ME			
Understand and manage our self-perception and choices.	Self-Compassion Combat insecurity by finding value within ourselves.	Self-Reflection Take responsibility for writing our own story.	Informed Decisiveness Make choices that align to our priorities.

An Overview of Allo Skills (other/you)

Allo skills are the foundation for relating to others. These skills help us respect our differences and create genuine connections. Allo skills allow us to release the responsibility of the thoughts, feelings, and behaviors of others. When we learn to use Allo skills, we confidently push our biases, assumptions, opinions, views, and judgment aside when interacting with kids and other adults. When we provide a space for kids and teens to safely express their needs where they genuinely feel valued and appreciated, they are capable of wellness. We also model healthy ways of engagement to prepare them for stepping into the "real world" on their own. Embedding this into our school environment is not only a fantastic learning opportunity for our kids, but also a tremendous gift to the future of humanity.

We've identified three Allo skills: Social Plasticity (Chapter 7), Empathetic Listening (Chapter 8), and Informed Responsiveness (Chapter 9).

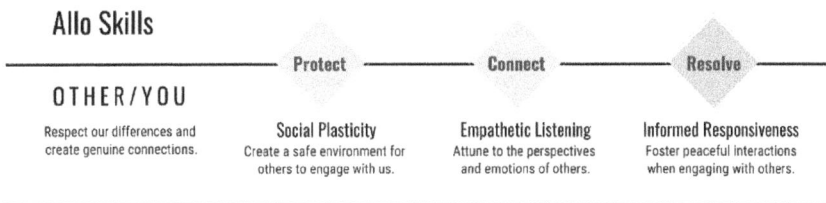

Allo Skills

	Protect	Connect	Resolve
OTHER/YOU Respect our differences and create genuine connections.	**Social Plasticity** Create a safe environment for others to engage with us.	**Empathetic Listening** Attune to the perspectives and emotions of others.	**Informed Responsiveness** Foster peaceful interactions when engaging with others.

An Overview of Ambi Skills (together/us)

Ambi skills are the foundation for forming partnerships and maintaining healthy relationships. Ambi skills help us break down barriers and work together toward a common goal. They enable us to create a safe space for people to come together so we can all express our opinions, feelings, needs, or ideas in a way that is clear, meaningful, and purposeful while still honoring one another. Ambi skills employ solution-focused tools to resolve disagreements reasonably, equitably, and effectively. We establish and maintain healthy boundaries, know our limits, and feel comfortable advocating for each other to ensure everyone feels heard, valued, and—at the very least—satisfied. Ultimately, the goal is to change unhealthy patterns to prevent (or repair) discord within relationships.

We've identified three Ambi skills: Relationship Reciprocity (Chapter 10), Compassionate Communication (Chapter 11), and Collaborative Resolution (Chapter 12.)

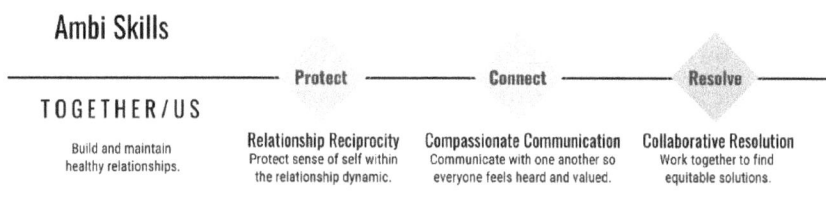

Ambi Skills

	Protect	Connect	Resolve
TOGETHER/US Build and maintain healthy relationships.	Relationship Reciprocity Protect sense of self within the relationship dynamic.	Compassionate Communication Communicate with one another so everyone feels heard and valued.	Collaborative Resolution Work together to find equitable solutions.

Getting the N.A.C. of It

To make the skills as easy as possible to implement, we broke them down into three steps:

Step 1. NOTICE. In every situation there is an opportunity to respond rather than react. The first step is noticing your current circumstances with curiosity rather than judgment.

Step 2. ASSESS. Assess if what you are currently doing is helpful or hurtful. Helpful means it is moving towards an effective resolution or is not doing additional harm to you or others. Hurtful means it has the potential of doing harm or isn't doing you or anyone else any good.

Step 3: CHOOSE. No matter what the situation is, you always have a choice. You can choose to stick to what you're doing, neutralize what you're doing, or reframe what you're doing.

We call this getting the N.A.C. of it.

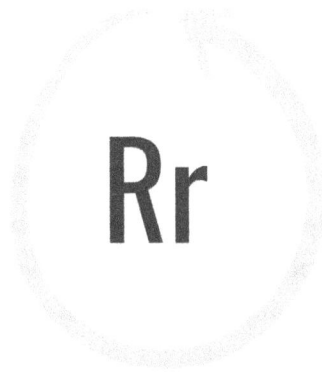

Rr

Rapid Resets

Getting the N.A.C. of it.

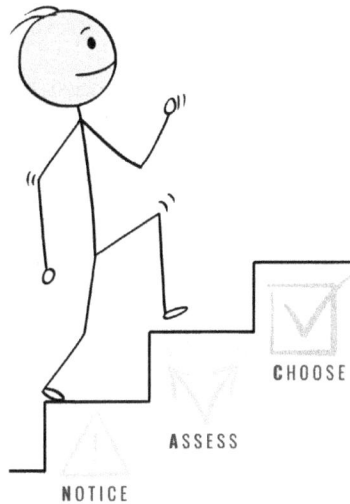

CHOOSE

ASSESS

NOTICE

Illustration by Cameron Caswell, TSC with ©zdeneksasek via Canva.com

Under each skill we have the choice to neutralize the experience and get back to baselines. We do this with Rapid Resets (see a full list of these in Appendix A). These are a curated collection of quick and easy techniques that we can use to turn off our amygdala's distress alarm and activate our parasympathetic nervous system. They tap into our basic senses to move our attention from our inner experience to our current surroundings. They can also help us shift the energy level from chaos to calm or expended to engaged.

The key to making rapid resets effective is selecting one proactively. Things to consider when choosing your go-to rapid reset:

1. Does it actually help me calm down? Counting to ten is a common calming technique; however, we've found that it doesn't actually work for most of our clients. No matter how popular a technique is, if it doesn't work for you, it's useless.

2. Can I use it within a wide range of circumstances? Many of our young clients use music to calm themselves down. Unfortunately, it's not a solution they can easily access in moments of high stress.

3. Am I comfortable using it? Perhaps taking deep breaths works for you and is easily accessible, but you feel like a dolt doing it in public. The last thing you need when you're feeling overwhelmed is to add embarrassment to the mix.

4. Am I willing to practice it regularly? When we're in the middle of an amygdala hijack, we're not in a state of mind to recall calming strategies—that takes rational thought. In order for rapid resets to be effective, they must be automatic responses. That means we must practice them often enough to hardwire them into our brain.

Do The Skills Need to be Taught in Order?

No. Although it's best to scaffold each of these skills from Auto to Allo and finally to Ambi skills, it's not necessary. It's more important to adapt to the specific needs and priorities of your school. For example, let's say you have data to show your school has a solid foundation of connectedness and a strong staff that can easily manage student behaviors, but they are ineffective at communicating with one another and solving problems. You may want to start by focusing on building proficiency in the Ambi skills. Or perhaps your staff put their heart and soul into student extracurriculars but have difficulty building bridges with parents. You may want to start building capacity in the Allo skills. The TSC framework is designed with ALL this in mind.

CHAPTER 4

~

Self-Compassion

*"You either walk inside your story and own it, or you stand
outside your story and hustle for your worthiness."*

–Brené Brown

There are many sources we can blame for the decline in mental health. Some favorites are social media, advertising, bullying, academic pressure, overscheduling, high expectations, virtual learning, social injustice, gun violence, the list goes on. There is one issue that we have seen at the center of all these problems: insecurity.

The Problem: Insecurity

Children absorb an endless stream of incoming messages telling them that they need to do more, be better, excel at everything. The push for high achievement and peak performance are well-intentioned. We've learned to associate benchmarks like straight A's with motivation, intelligence, mental well-being, and other desirable qualities. Conversely, lackluster performance such as poor grades create the illusion of laziness, incompetency, and mental instability. Although in reality grades and other measures of achievement provide little to no insight into our character, capabilities, or mental health, we continue to enforce the message that our self-worth is measured by our performance. When children inevitably fall short of these expectations, their inner dialogue becomes more self-critical and judgmental. The more they try to "fix" themselves in order to be accepted by their parents, their educators, and society overall. Psychologists theorize that when children feel insecure about being accepted by their parents and the adults around them, they feel lost, alone, and anxious.[28] [29] In other words, insecure.

Once formed, this belief that we are not good enough becomes the filter through which we experience the world. The more we feel we have to fake who we are to get the validation we crave, the more insecure we become in who we are and our right to be unconditionally loved. It's a filter too many of us carry as we transition into adulthood.

This belief is reflected in our fixation on accumulating friends and likes on social media. Because our culture celebrates being "more"— more fit, more attractive, more healthy, wealthier, more followers, more likes—we feel pressured to carefully curate the version of us we share with the world. We repress our authentic selves out of fear of rejection and ridicule[30] and settle for the superficial acceptance and fleeting approval our fake selves earn.

This disingenuous facade can seep into our real lives as well. Many of us, especially our vulnerable youth, believe we have to choose between being liked and being ourselves. We end up becoming people

---

[28] Bowlby, J. (1973). Attachment and Loss, Vol. 2: Separation, Anxiety, and Anger. New York: Basic Books.

[29] Ainsworth, M., Blehar, M., Waters, E., & Wall, S. (1978). Patterns of Attachment. Hillsdale, NJ: Erlbaum.

[30] May, R. (2009). Man's search for himself. WW Norton & Company

pleasers and dangerously more concerned about living up to others' expectations than our own.[31]

Why It Matters

There is a wealth of research that links low self-esteem and insecurity to poor academic performance, depression, aggression, bullying, cutting, delinquency, violence, and other mental and behavioral problems.[32] [33] Self-esteem is also vital to our success as adults. Lack of it results in depression, increased absenteeism, lower productivity, relationship problems, and drug and alcohol use, to name a few. We are no longer able to function with stability in the world on both a physical and emotional basis.[34]

The Current Solution: The Self Improvement Movement

The current solution to feeling better about ourselves is improving ourselves. We constantly strive to measure up to cultural norms, religious convictions, and societal expectations. We just need to be thinner, fitter, stronger, smarter, richer. We're led to believe that at the end of the race we'll find happiness, self-esteem, fulfillment, wealth, and peace. If we don't have those things, clearly it's because we aren't trying hard enough.

---

[31] Gilligan, C., Rogers, A. G., & Noel, N. (2018). Cartography of a Lost Time: Mapping the Crisis of Connection. In C. Gilligan, N. Way, A. Ali, & P. Noguera (Eds.), The Crisis of Connection: Roots, Consequences, and Solutions (pp. 65–87). NYU Press

[32] Keegan, 1987; Branden, 1994; Frank, 1996; Candito, J.,1996; Donnellan, 2005; Marsh, 2005; Robins, 2005; Rosenthal, 2005.

[33] Cision PR Newswire provided by Dove (2016)

[34] van den Bos (2009)

We're teaching this to our children, too. We push them to practice more, take harder classes, get better grades, and never mess up.

One of our young clients, Clarissa, came to us to help her manage her anxiety. During our introductory session, we asked her to tell us three things she liked about herself. She struggled to come up with even one. Then we asked her to describe herself. Without hesitation she spouted off a list as if from memory: "I'm lazy, I'm an ADHD kid so I'm a bad student, I get in trouble a lot..." She finished by explaining that she was trying really hard to be better, but she was struggling to make changes. She had concluded that she couldn't do anything right. She was unhappy with who she was.

Why It's Not Solving the Problem

The relentless pressure that we must change to feel better about ourselves is making us feel worse. It sends the message that who we are right now isn't OK. This is why taking responsibility for our mistakes, even small ones, may make us feel like a major failure. Our instinct is to deny, hide, or lie about our actions in an attempt to "save face" and protect our fragile sense of self-worth.

Rather than feeling motivated and energized to explore new interests and talents, we feel burdened to fix what's wrong with us. No matter how much we do, we never seem to get to a place where happiness and fulfillment are within reach. We often give up even trying.

The TSC Solution: Self-Compassion

Before we can start doing *more*, it's important to feel OK with ourselves right here, right now. We can do this by creating a safe space for ourselves and learning to see the value of who we are in the moment. This is called Self-Compassion.

Self-Compassion

PURPOSE: Protect sense of self.
HOW: Separate WHO from DO.

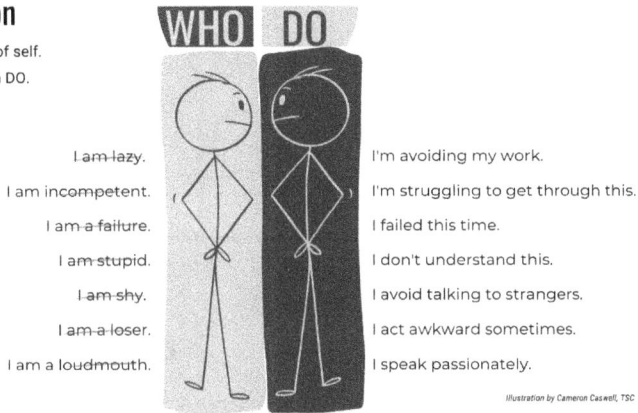

WHO | DO

I am lazy. | I'm avoiding my work.
I am incompetent. | I'm struggling to get through this.
I am a failure. | I failed this time.
I am stupid. | I don't understand this.
I am shy. | I avoid talking to strangers.
I am a loser. | I act awkward sometimes.
I am a loudmouth. | I speak passionately.

Illustration by Cameron Caswell, TSC

Self-Compassion protects our sense of self by separating WHO we are from what we DO. It's the difference between being a liar and telling a lie or being a loser and losing a game. This distinction may seem small, but it makes an enormous difference in how we perceive ourselves.

When we blame our faults, mistakes, and shortcomings on WHO we are, we perceive our character as irrevocably flawed. If we view our failures as evidence that we are inadequate or defective, we relinquish any hope of overcoming them. We get trapped in a wheel of self-defeat:

Wheel of Self-Defeat

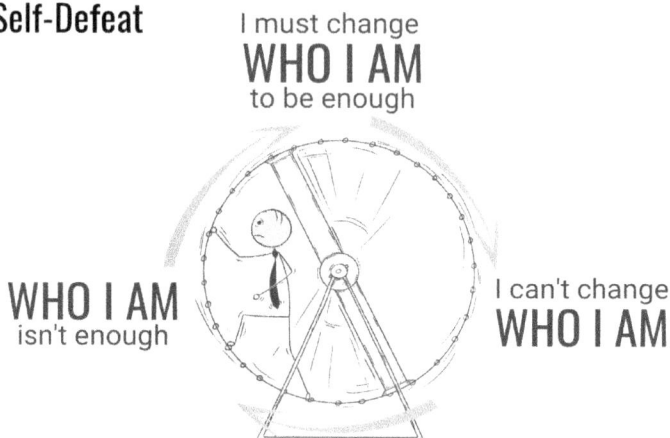

I must change
WHO I AM
to be enough

WHO I AM
isn't enough

I can't change
WHO I AM

Illustration by Cameron Caswell, TSC with @zdeneksasek via Canva.com

We start to believe that if people knew who we really were, they wouldn't accept us. To counter this, we learn to hide our true selves from others, sometimes even from ourselves.

Self-Compassion is built upon the understanding that our value far surpasses what we DO (or don't do.) It allows us to accept that we are imperfect beings trying to do the best we can under the current circumstances and with the resources and knowledge that we have at the time. This doesn't give us permission to shirk responsibility or behave badly. It gives us the freedom to take accountability for our actions and make amends without shame. When we acknowledge that we make mistakes, we don't become our mistakes, we are released from the wheel of self-defeat. When we no longer measure our self-worth by our ability to meet expectations, we feel empowered to overcome challenges and pursue personal growth with enthusiasm and a true sense of fulfillment.

Getting the N.A.C. of It

Step 1: NOTICE you need Self-Compassion

NOTICE

When we feel out-of-sorts or outright bad about ourselves, chances are what we're DOING doesn't align with WHO we are or aspire to be. Perhaps we feel bad because we made a mistake or hurt someone. We could be thinking things like, "if people knew who I really was they wouldn't like me" or "I'm not smart enough to figure that out." We may simply feel queasy or have a sense that we're in trouble, but have no idea why. All of these are clues that we're tangling up WHO you are with what you DO. Simply acknowledge that. Remember to notice with curiosity, not criticism.

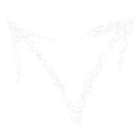

Step 2: ASSESS if it's helpful or hurtful

ASSESS

If our belief about WHO we are sparks positive change from a place of choice and empowerment, it is helpful. If it pushes us into a pit of despair and self-loathing, they are hurtful. A good clue that your perception of WHO you are is hurtful is the word "should." I *should* be more generous. I *should* be more motivated. This indicates that we feel like we need to change WHO we are in order to be *enough*. "Shoulds" like this can push us to the brink of feeling burdened and resentful.[35] That's when they become hurtful.

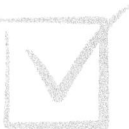

Step 3: CHOOSE what to do next

CHOOSE

Once you notice how you view WHO you are and have determined if it's helpful or hurtful, you can choose what to do about it.

---

[35] Oh et al. (2020)

Choice #1: Stick with it

You have the choice to continue doing exactly what you've been doing, and you can already predict the outcome. If the outcome is what you want, great. If it's not, just realize that by choosing not to change, there is little chance the outcome will either.

Choice #2: Neutralize it

If it's inappropriate to express the full extent of the emotion you're feeling without consequences, or you prefer to deal with it privately at a later time, you can neutralize your emotions with Rapid Resets.

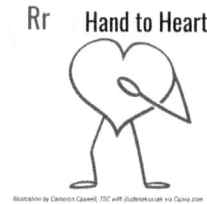

Rr   Hand to Heart

Illustration by Catherin Caswell, TSC with studentsu.uk via Canva.com

This one is a therapeutic technique used with variations such as putting a hand to your forehead or your stomach or using your left versus right hand.[36] The effects are there with any of these, so let's keep it simple and just place one of your hands over your heart. Sit, stand, or lay down comfortably. You can close your eyes, look down at the floor, or find a focal point such as a picture on the wall. The goal is to attune to your body responses when feeling even the slightest distress so you can protect yourself from spiraling too deeply into despair, which is difficult to move out of. Notice where you're feeling strain, and picture untangling that for relief. Try to bring your breath to an in-through-the-nose and out-through-the-mouth pattern, at a slow, steady pace. With your hand still gently but firmly placed over your heart, pay attention to any discomfort you feel in your body. Envision that unraveling. You can add in some reassuring words to remind yourself of your strengths. Tell yourself that you deserve freedom from being stuck in this moment and will move out of it when you're ready to take that step. You can use this anytime you need to self-soothe.

Choice #3: Reframe it
When we separate WHO we are from what we DO, we allow for self-forgiveness and change. In order to realign what we DO with WHO we are or aspire to be, we can recast ourselves as the hero of our own story. A fun yet highly effective way to see ourselves as the hero is by turning our perceived weaknesses into strengths or superpowers. Often the very things that make us feel victimized and powerless are our biggest strengths in disguise. Superheroes have been mesmerizing us with their powers for decades. But when you dig into their backstories, you learn that even the invincible struggled to control their powers when they first discovered them.

In Smallville, Clark Kent accidentally sets his classroom on fire when his heat ray vision is triggered for the first time. After a few more

---

[36] Dr. Kristin Neff, https://self-compassion.org/#

embarrassing fire faux pas, he learns how to control it.[37] And who can forget Peter Parker face planting into the billboard sign the first time he tried swinging from his web.[38] But he kept trying and in no time was flying through the streets of NYC.

The point is, superpowers aren't always super at first. In fact, they can be quite mortifying. The secret is learning to acknowledge what they are and learn to use them to help yourself and others. We did this with Clarissa, the youth with ADHD discussed earlier in this chapter. A large portion of her story spiraled around her being an "ADHD kid." Her beliefs about what she could do, perceptions of how people treated her, and reactions to others were all in response to feeling she was broken and doomed for a life of struggle. While it's true that ADHD adds barriers to excelling in a traditional school setting, in other venues, it can serve as a superpower. We helped Clarissa recast herself as the hero of her story by turning her perceived weaknesses into strengths. Because of the way her brain worked, she was highly creative, could get laser-focused on something she was passionate about, and extended empathy to others.

Here are some more examples of how perceived weaknesses can be transformed into superpowers:

Old Weakness	New Superpower
Bossy	Assertive
Impatient	Passionate
Indecisive	Easy going
Shy	Introspective
Stubborn	Determined

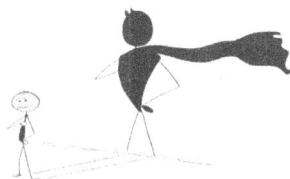

Illustration by Cameron Caswell, TSC with @zdeneksasek via Canva.com

Once we reframe our weaknesses into superpowers, they not only become lighter, but we can harness their strengths to propel us higher.

---

[37] Smallville. (2022). Season 2, ep. 2

[38] Spider-Man (2002)

The Biggest Takeaways

1. The key to Self-Compassion is separating WHO you are from what you DO.
2. We get trapped on the Wheel of Self-Defeat when we believe our self-worth is dependent on changing who we are to meet expectations.
3. We can reframe our perceived weaknesses as superpowers to become the hero of our own story.

CHAPTER 5

~

Self-Reflection

*"If we could change ourselves, the tendencies in the world
would also change. As a man changes his own nature,
so does the attitude of the world change towards him."*

-Ghandi

For the majority of our 200,000 years on Earth,[39] our instinct to constantly scan our surroundings for dangers protected us from wild beasts and treacherous environments. The most attuned to these perils survived. Over time, this hardwired humans to pay more attention to negative things and overlook positive ones.

The Problem: Negative Self-Talk

Thanks to modern conveniences, many of us aren't confronted with life-threatening situations on a daily basis anymore. Even so, our brain's first priority is still survival. The busy, hectic lifestyle so many of us celebrate creates an endless parade of stressors which our brain perceives

---

[39] 2.2 million if you count other Homo species. Or base it on your belief of human creation.

as danger. In response, it floods our body with a steady stream of stress hormones. These compromise our ability to think rationally about our negatively skewed thoughts and make it difficult to regulate the emotions and behaviors they spark.

Let's say you're walking down the hall and spot a colleague coming towards you. You smile and wave at them. They give you a quick glance then walk past you without even a nod of acknowledgement. You immediately think, "They must be mad at me. What did I do wrong?" You start racking your brain trying to remember the last time you interacted with them and what you possibly could have done that warranted such a callous blow off. Even though you can't think of anything, you're sure it must have been really bad. You worry that you've ruined the relationship. When you arrive home your child is upset because the fruit snacks are all gone. You think, "Everyone expects so much from me, and all I do is let them down." You snap at your child, "How did you get to be so spoiled? You should be thankful for all the food you have."

When we allow our feelings to occupy the driver's seat, we end up reacting to what we perceive others are doing to us. It's difficult to feel in control of our own lives when we feel like we're at the constant mercy of who and what is around us.

Feeling like we don't have control over what happens to us also takes a considerable physical and emotional toll on us. It causes increased tension in our body and negatively impacts our behavior. Common responses are "snapping" or getting angry very quickly, unexpected mood swings, and screaming or yelling at loved ones.[40] It has also been shown that educators experience a spike in stress when they feel like

[40] American Psychological Association (2020)

their classroom demands exceed their resources for coping.[41] This is why we tend to react emotionally and impulsively. Here's a story we heard from a female vice principal:

After working at an elementary school for two years and all signs pointing towards becoming the next principal, the job went to someone else. Someone younger. A man. I tried to go with the flow, but I was resentful. Then I started to notice an increasing number of inequities across the district. I got angrier by the day. My once sunny disposition became negative, and I started to "lose my shit" at work (a.k.a. yelling at staff). These hurtful emotions started seeping into my personal life, too. My patience was shot. At one point, my daughter made an offhand comment about how the lights on our Christmas tree looked crooked. This little criticism agitated me so much that I picked the tree up and threw it over the balcony. Here I am, trained to maintain a secure learning environment for hundreds of kids, completely out of control. Now that I can reflect objectively about my behaviors, I know I could have handled them a lot better. I also understand that at the time, I was stuck in a state of fight or flight, which compromised my ability to think rationally. I know it's not an excuse, but it is an explanation.

Reactive behavior can be so subtle that we don't even realize we're reacting at all. Perhaps a student makes a snarky remark when you ask them to stop talking. You feel like they're challenging your authority. You make a sarcastic comment back that you later regret. Maybe a stranger bumps into you on a crowded sidewalk and you mumble under your breath (but loud enough for them to hear), "Some people are just so rude."

---

[41] Mccarthy et al (2015)

Why It Matters

Although reactive behaviors give us the illusion of power and regaining control, they often end up making the situation worse. We risk escalating conflict, ruining relationships, and piling on a new source of guilt that further compromises our own well-being.

Yet repressing these feelings lead to headaches, stomachaches, insomnia, anxiety, depression, and other health problems. Bottled up emotions also makes it harder to refrain from acting out the next time. This is especially common in children because their emotional responses are still maturing. However, adults have been known to throw a temper tantrum or two when things don't go their way.

The Current Solution: Self-Regulation

So what do we do when we can't sit still or focus when we're bored? How do we stop ourselves from yelling or punching the wall when we're angry or smile pleasantly even when we're feeling miserable inside? Psychologists have been trying to noodle that one through for decades. The leading theory centers on self-regulation. This states that if we are not happy with our behavior, we can correct it by building new pathways in the brain[42] [43] [44] to behave in

---

[42] In the 1970s, Albert Bandura introduced Social Learning Theory claiming "most human behavior is learned observationally through modeling: from observing others one forms an idea of how new behaviors are performed, and on later occasions, this coded information serves as a guide for action." He later added that "humans are able to control their behavior through a process known as self-regulation." This grew into self-regulation theory (SRT), which is based on the idea that much of our behavior is directed toward accomplishing goals. According to modern SRT expert Roy Baumeisterour behavior is determined by our personal standards of good behavior, our motivation to meet those standards, the degree to which we are consciously aware of our circumstances and our actions, and the extent of our willpower to resist temptations and choose the best path.

[43] Bandura (1991)

[44] Baumeister & Vohs (2007)

ways deemed more socially appropriate, regardless of our internal thoughts and emotions.[45]

Strategies for regulating our behaviors, emotions, and thoughts include things like using reward systems, thinking positively, avoiding triggers, decreasing risk factors, meditating, and practicing mindfulness.[46] Whichever the strategy, greater self-regulation is positively correlated with well-being[47] including greater life satisfaction, stronger social support, and more positive feelings.[48] This is why we continue implementing these approaches.

Why It's Not Solving the Problem

One core problem we encounter with self-regulation strategies is that it still puts the primary focus on behavioral modification—only now we're expected to control ourselves rather than being externally controlled. In the end, it boils down to trying to change our external self to appease others. In the end, it boils down to trying to change our external self to appease others. That is why it's easy to misinterpret an outward appearance of acquiescence and composure as internal resolution. What we've seen in the children with whom we work is that they learn to repress how they truly think and feel, their genuine selves, in order to be liked and accepted. Self-regulation becomes more about pleasing others and removing their discomfort than addressing one's own discomfort and needs.

Trying to suppress or repress our thoughts or emotions doesn't make them go away. That's because what we resist persists. In his well-known "white bear" study,[49] social psychologist Dr. Daniel Wegner

---

[45] Stosny (2011)

[46] Razza et al. (2013)

[47] Skowron et al. (2003)

[48] Verzeletti et al. (2016)

[49] Wegner et al. (1987)

found that when we try to suppress a thought (don't yawn or don't think of a white bear) our brain is compelled to "check in" to make sure we're obeying the command. Ironically, in order to confirm we're not thinking about something, we have to first think about it. So, the more we try to repress a thought or emotion, the more likely it is to appear.

Not all negative thoughts are bad and not all positive thoughts are good-these techniques don't account for that. Negative thoughts such as "This relationship is toxic," "I'm worried," or "I'm uncomfortable," can provide important intel to help us make more informed decisions. Overriding these negative thoughts with positive ones such as, "Don't worry, be happy," "Stay calm, and carry on," and "Look on the bright side," may repress them, not make them go away. If we reject, deny, or gloss over something serious that needs to be addressed, we may end up self-talking ourselves into staying in an abusive relationship, holding on to an unhealthy habit, or putting ourselves in a dangerous situation.

The same can be said about emotions. Our uncomfortable emotions are not only valid, but they are also powerful agents of security, clarity, and change. Anger can protect us from exploitation, injustice, and assault. It can motivate us to problem-solve, overcome obstacles, and give us the courage we need to take control of a scary situation. Fear heightens our awareness and prepares us to flee. It's also a sign that we are pushing ourselves outside our comfort zone.

Additionally, it takes substantial work, practice, and effort (e.g., self-regulation) in order to use self-regulation techniques. Therefore, the people who most need self-regulation skills are the least equipped to use them. For example, the more impulsive we are, the more self-control we need to inhibit it. The more we struggle to avoid "bad behavior," the more we deplete our willpower and motivation to resist temptations and urges.[50] It becomes yet another thing we should do, but fail to do because it's too hard.

---

[50] Wagner et al. (2013)

The TSC Solution: Self-Reflection

Self-reflection is a way to understand our own thoughts, emotions, and behaviors in unison and learn to align them with our priorities. We do this using the Story Spiral.

Self-Reflection

PURPOSE: Connect to self.
HOW: Rewrite your story.

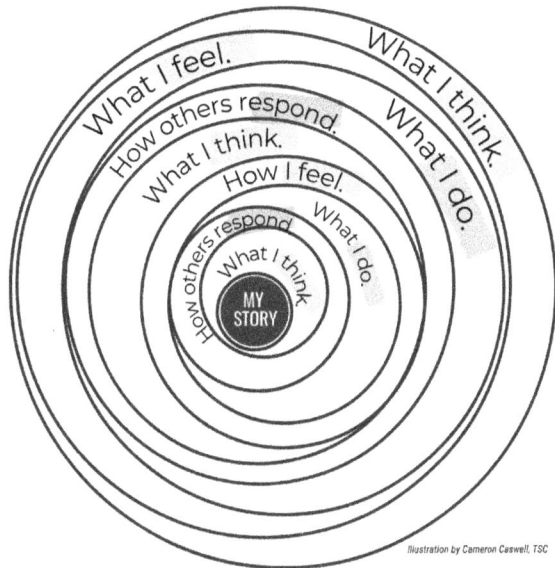

Illustration by Cameron Caswell, TSC

Our Story Spiral

The concept of the Story Spiral is built upon the belief that our thoughts, emotions, and behaviors are tightly interwoven and impact one another in a fluid, multi-directional chain reaction. How they interplay with one another influences what we notice and how we interact with it. This ultimately impacts how we experience the world. The story spiral is built upon two key concepts:

We see what we believe: There is far too much sensory input around us for our brain to process without becoming overloaded. So it hones in on a smaller subset of information it deems important and filters out the rest. Think of it like having our own search algorithm that's always looking for evidence to support what we already believe. This means, at any given time, we are magnifying aspects of a situation that align with our story and filtering out or reinterpreting the ones that do not. If you believe you're disliked, you may notice a curt response or dismissive look and completely miss a kind smile or invitation to join a conversation. This is why you and I can both be in the same situation and yet have completely different experiences.

We get what we expect: There is quite a buzz around the power of the mind. Positive thinking. Manifestation. Visualization. Limiting beliefs. Can our thoughts really manipulate our reality? Yes and no. Thoughts don't change what happens around us and to us. Thoughts change our story spiral, which impacts how we react to a situation, which in turn influences the results of that situation. When we focus our attention on an expectation, our brain is constantly looking for a solution just like an app running in the background. This is known as confirmation bias[51]. If we tell our brain that we're going to fail, our subconscious mind starts looking for ways to ensure we fail. If we tell our brain we're going to succeed, it looks for ways to set ourselves up for success. We haven't manipulated the world around us, but we have manipulated how we experience it.

To understand your story spiral, ask, "What is the story I'm telling myself?" We use the word "story" because it implies that it is a product of our imagination. It's not reality but rather one of many possible versions of an experience. It opens the possibility for other versions and gives us space to rewrite our story. Based on your story, fill in the story spiral. Once you are aware of what is creating your story spiral you can start to change it. Sometimes all it takes is changing just one thread

---

[51] Guiney, P., W. Goodfellow, AND Timothy J. Canfield. An Overview of Confirmation Bias in Science: Examples and Opportunities for Improvement. Society of Environmental Toxicology and Chemistry (SETAC) SCICON2 – SETAC North America 41st Annual Meeting, N/A, N/A, November 15 - 19, 2020.

(e.g., withdraw from everyone), to cause the whole thing to unravel.

Remember the story above about the colleague who ignored you in the hallway? There are an unlimited number of story spirals you could follow:

Story Spiral #1: I'm not likable.

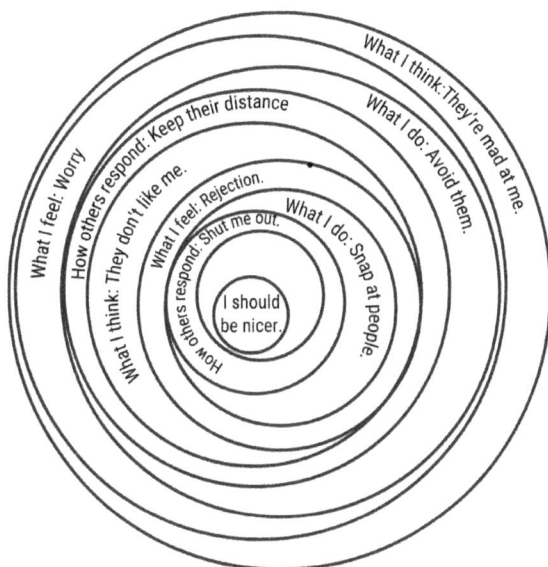

+ What I think: They're mad at me. I must have done something wrong.
+ What I feel: Worry.
+ What I do: Avoid people.
+ How others respond: Keep their distance.
+ What I think: My coworkers don't like me.
+ How I feel: Rejection.
+ What I do: Snap at people.
+ How others respond: They shut me out.

Story Spiral #2: My coworkers aren't friendly.

+ What I think: They're being rude.
+ How I feel: Annoyance.
+ What I do: Give them the brush off next time you see them.
+ How others respond: Say something snarky.
+ What I think: I shouldn't care what they think of me.
+ How I feel: Resentful.
+ What I do: Accuse them of being a snob.
+ How others respond: Snub me.

Story Spiral #3: My colleagues are awesome.

+ What I think: They are so focused on their thoughts they didn't see me.
+ What I feel: Amusement.
+ What I do: Seek them out later to catch up.
+ How others respond: Appreciate me.
+ What I think: I'm grateful to work with these people.
+ What I feel: Contentment.
+ What I do: Interact more with your colleagues.
+ How they respond: Engage with me more.

Getting the N.A.C. of It

NOTICE

Step 1: NOTICE you need self-reflection
Before we can self-reflect, we must notice that we're telling ourselves a story. For example, what story did we tell ourselves when our colleague passed us in the hallway? Remember to notice with curiosity, not criticism.

Step 2: ASSESS if it's helpful or hurtful

Rather than analyzing each thought, emotion, and reaction individually, we can reflect on if they're forming a story spiral that is helpful or hurtful.

ASSESS

Helpful story spirals lead to solutions and insight. They provide us with a roadmap for resolution and motivate us to make amends and instigate change. Helpful stories focus on what we can control.

Hurtful story spirals entrench us in unsolvable problems and rob us of agency and self-determination. They paralyze us and compel us to hide and deny. Often a hurtful story spiral starts because we confuse thoughts with facts and emotions with personal characteristics.

Hurtful story spirals are also based on a perception that what happens to us is controlled by outside forces, luck, or fate. Someone made us angry. Some event ruined our day. Everything would be better if so-and-so changed. Although it may provide us an excuse for shirking responsibility and accountability for what happens to us, these stories put us in a victim mentally. They overwhelm us and make us feel powerless.

Step 3: CHOOSE what to do next

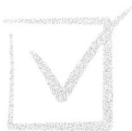

Accepting responsibility for our actions requires courage, self-awareness, and a belief that we can learn to do better.

CHOOSE

Choice 1: Stick with it

You have the choice to continue doing exactly what you've been doing, and you can already predict the outcome. If the outcome is what you want, great. If it's not, just realize that by choosing not to change, there is little chance the outcome will either.

Choice 2: Neutralize it

We can use Rapid Resets to pull ourselves out of a hurtful story spiral long enough to give our body a chance to calm down, bring our rational brain back online, and bring our energy back to baseline.

Rr   Thumb Drum

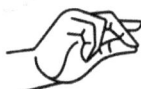

Illustration by Cameron Caswell, TSC with @StampArt via Canva.com

This is a great technique to use if you need to raise your energy, such as when you're feeling unmotivated or sluggish, or lower your energy, such as when you're feeling antsy or anxious. You can do this without anyone knowing about it, which is why we love Thumb Drum for those who want to be discrete.

Take either hand and bring each of your fingers to your thumb. Change the pressure as needed, depending on whether you need to get extra energy out (add pressure) or whether you need to go from chaos to calm (lighten the pressure). You can also quicken the pace moving from finger to finger if you need to increase your energy level. You can slow down the pace if you need to decrease your energy level.

Choice 3: Reframe it

If we feel powerless, it's often because we're letting others control our narrative. We may be letting them determine our worth, dictate how we feel, and decide what happens to us. If we want to change our reality, we need to rewrite our story.

An easy way to rewrite our story is to replace our "*shoulds*" with "*coulds*." *Should* implies shortcomings: If I were a good/smart/competent person I would be doing THIS, but I'm not doing THIS, so

WHO I am must be bad/stupid/inept. Because *should* assumes that WHO we are is defective, it crushes our self-esteem and motivation.

The simple fix to this *shoulding* problem is replacing "sh" with "c." Instead of saying, "I *should* do this," say, "I *could* do this." While *should* keep us stuck, *could* gives us choice. *Could* assumes that WHO we are strives to DO the best we can, but we don't always succeed. If we don't feel like we did our best, *could* gives us room to explore why with curiosity rather than criticism and paves the way to make informed decisions (see chapter 6).

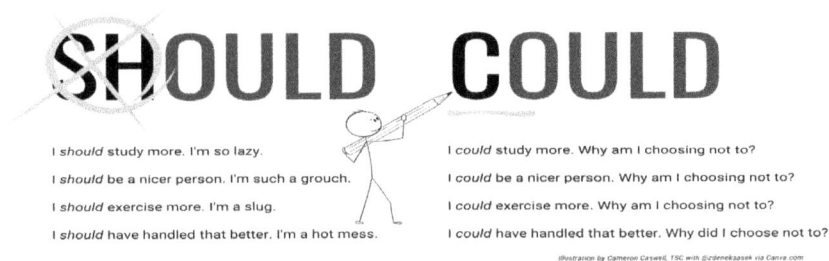

I *should* study more. I'm so lazy.	I *could* study more. Why am I choosing not to?
I *should* be a nicer person. I'm such a grouch.	I *could* be a nicer person. Why am I choosing not to?
I *should* exercise more. I'm a slug.	I *could* exercise more. Why am I choosing not to?
I *should* have handled that better. I'm a hot mess.	I *could* have handled that better. Why did I choose not to?

Illustration by Cameron Caswell, TSC with @zdenekkasek via Canva.com

Stepping up and taking responsibility for our own story is one of the most empowering things we can do. It's also one of the hardest when things get tough. There will always be extenuating circumstances that impact us, sometimes in a traumatic and debilitating way. Taking responsibility doesn't mean shouldering the blame for other people's actions, it means acknowledging that there is always something we *could* do. It's also not forgetting or pretending our missteps never happened; it's about learning from our experiences and defining a more constructive way that we move forward.

The Biggest Takeaways

1. Our story spirals are shaped by how our thoughts, emotions, and actions interplay with one another.

2. Accepting responsibility for our actions requires courage, self-awareness, and a belief that we can learn to do better.

3. The next time you feel the shaming *"should"* about to roll off your tongue, remember you *could* say *"could"* instead.

CHAPTER 6

~

Informed Decisiveness

"Everything can be taken from a man but one thing:
the last of the human freedoms—to choose one's attitude in
any given set of circumstances, to choose one's own way."

- Victor Frankel[52]

W here are you reading this? Why here? Why now? Are you aware of the long series of decisions you had to make to arrive at this very moment? Probably not.

The Problem: Mindless Decision-Making

Although everything we do involves making choices, we make most of them automatically with little effort or thinking. We'd never get anything done if we didn't. It's been estimated that an average person makes 35,000 remotely conscious choices per day[53] (226.7 of those are just about food[54]). Assuming we get seven hours of sleep every night,

---

[52] Frankl (1962)
[53] Sahakian & Labuzetta, 2013
[54] Wansink and Sobal, 2007

that means we are making roughly one decision every two seconds, and educators make around 1,500 daily decisions in the classroom alone.[55]

In today's fast-paced world, it's not surprising we feel overwhelmed by all the decisions we have to make. Our brain's prefrontal cortex, which is responsible for decision-making, can only process so much information at once. To prevent it from being overloaded by simple routine tasks and be able to process complex choices as quickly and effortlessly as possible, our brain creates cognitive shortcuts, known as heuristics.[56] A majority of our choices are made subconsciously,[57] relying heavily on intuition, emotions, memories, biases, and immediate rewards. Studies suggest that making decisions based on immediate rewards in particular can lead to chronic stress[58] which in turn impedes our ability to think objectively and rationally, which leads to more poor decision-making.

On the flip side, we may agonize for hours over some decisions, analyzing every option, outcome, and datapoint we can find. This often happens when we have too many choices (e.g., sixty choices of toothpaste), have a lot weighing on the result of our choice (e.g. where you end up living for the next ten years), don't trust our decision-making ability, or are scared of how other people will respond to our decisions. In these situations, we feel so overwhelmed that we end up choosing the direction of our lives based on internal impulse or external influences. Or we simply do nothing at all.

In either extreme, our choices are often made in a state of oblivion or panic that leads us blindly down a path we haven't selected.

---

[55] https://www.edutopia.org/blog/battling-decision-fatigue-gravity-goldberg-renee-houser

[56] Bobadilla-suarez S, Love BC. Fast or frugal, but not both: Decision heuristics under time pressure. J Exp Psychol Learn Mem Cogn. 2018;44(1):24-33. doi:10.1037/xlm0000419

[57] Kahneman, Daniel (2011). Thinking Fast and Slow

[58] https://www.frontiersin.org/articles/10.3389/fnbeh.2020.00081/full

Why It Matters

The problem with making too many decisions subconsciously, or by default, is that we lose control over what happens to us. Self-help guru Tony Robbins[59] coined this "The Niagara Syndrome" because when we get swept up in the current of life (current events, current fears, current challenges) all we can focus on is navigating around the perilous rocks in front of us (AKA the short-term problems). We end up drifting into the life we have rather than choosing the life we want.

When we forgo making decisions, we no longer feel in control over our own lives. Martin Seligman demonstrated this phenomenon, called "learned helplessness," in his classic 1967 experiment. He placed dogs in a chamber which triggered an electric shock when they tried to escape. After a period of time, the dogs gave up trying. Even when the shock was removed, they still didn't try. They had developed a belief that they were powerless. Seligman speculated that when humans experience a series of negative events without having any perceived control we no longer believe that we can influence what happens to us or around us. We give up trying.[60]

How do we break out of this trap of indecisiveness? Studies suggest that we can improve the quality of our lives simply by becoming more competent at making decisions.[61] The good news is, decision-making is an art that can be learned.

The Current Solution: Decision-Making Tools

There certainly is no shortage of decision-making strategies and tools: analytical decision-making, absolute or autocratic decision making,

---

[59] Awaken the Giant Within

[60] Seligman, M., Maier, S.F., & Geer, J.H. (1968). Alleviation of learned helplessness in the dog. Journal of abnormal psychology, 73 3, 256-62.

[61] https://www.cmu.edu/news/archive/2007/May/may17_decision.shtml

autonomous decision making, collaborative decision-making, command decision-making, consensus-based decision-making, simple feature decision-making...you get the picture. With so many decision-making tools, how do we choose?

What It's Not Solving the Problem

Each decision-making tool provides a step-by-step process to help us select between different alternatives based on facts, figures, data, and research. They all rely heavily on logic, awareness, rationality, and objectivity. Although it seems logical to implement a structured framework, most of the time it's not practical. This type of complex and effortful thinking requires attention, motivation, and self-control,[62] resources that are limited and quickly depleted when we are already busy, stressed, and tired. Ironically, the stressful process of decision making in and of itself can drain us of the resources we need to make a good decision. That means the more important it is to make a good decision, the harder it is to make a good decision.

This is why we rely heavily on more easily accessible information like intuition, emotions, memories, biases, and immediate rewards[63] to make our decisions. This is often referred to as our subconscious or "gut instinct." Even when we do take the time to systematically walk through a rational decision-making process, we are subconsciously swayed by our internal beliefs, emotions and bias.

Experts suggest that we counter these negative influences by taking a beat before we make a decision and notice what thoughts and emotions automatically surface.[64] We love this concept, but we also know when we're stressed/tired/overwhelmed/etc., by the time we remember to take a pause, we've already made the decision. That creates quite a conundrum.

---

[62] Kahneman, Daniel (2011). Thinking Fast and Slow
[63] https://www.ncbi.nlm.nih.gov/pmc/articles/PMC5346059/
[64] Cleaning-Your-Mental-Mess-Scientifically

The TSC Solution: Informed Decisiveness

Rather than trying to override our auto response system, let's intentionally reprogram it. We call this informed decisiveness. Rather than fighting our instinct to make decisions by default, informed decisiveness enables us to design the framework that informs our default mode. It starts by defining our values, priorities, ethical codes, and goals as precisely and succinctly as we can. We call these guideposts. These allow us to make choices that strengthen our sense of self and well-being.

Informed Decisiveness

PURPOSE: Resolve personal choices.
HOW: Guideposts.

Is this the **KIND HONEST HELPFUL** thing to do?

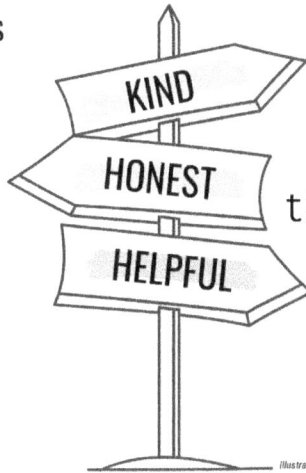

Illustration by Cameron Caswell, TSC

Here's a list of ten common guideposts:

1. Happiness
2. Health
3. Honesty
4. Justice
5. Kindness
6. Service
7. Stability
8. Success
9. Wealth
10. Work Ethic

When our guideposts are clear and accessible, we are able to make decisions quickly, even effortlessly, that align with who we aspire to be and where we want to go. Guideposts keep us moving towards the best version of ourselves. It's like picking out a hiking trail. First you decide where you want to hike to, then you find the best path to get you there. As you hike, you can look out for guideposts to make sure you're sticking to the path you chose. These guideposts give us the information we need to make optimal decisions even when we're not our optimal selves.

When we use clear guideposts, we feel capable and confident in our ability to make decisions rapidly that will align with WHO we are and what we strive to DO. When we align WHO we are and what we DO, we reduce internal conflict. Even when our choices do not result in the outcome we expected, because they were based on our guideposts, we don't feel the need to beat ourselves up for making a mistake. We can learn from it instead.

One of our clients, Asa, was extremely upset by her son Malik's poor grades, lying, and cheating. She had taken away his phone, grounded

him from seeing friends, and banned him from playing video games. Nothing seemed to work. In fact, he was simply becoming angrier and more deceitful. Asa didn't understand why Malik was behaving this way. He was smart enough to get straight A's if he would only try harder. When we talked to Malik we got a different perspective. He believed that all that mattered to his mom was that he got good grades so he could get into a good school. He felt like she was constantly on him about it. But he was struggling to stay focused and even care about his classes. So he started cheating to make sure he kept his grades up. He didn't see what the problem was. He was giving Asa what she asked for. In fact, he was angry at her for telling him one thing and then yelling at him because he didn't do it the way she wanted. So he just lied to keep her off his back. We worked with Asa to define what was most important to her. It turned out that it wasn't grades, even though her actions made it seem that way. It was more important to her to develop a strong relationship with Malik and help him see his potential. She realized that the choices she had been making weren't aligned with her priorities and started making changes in how she interacted with her son. That made all the difference.

Informed decisiveness also gives us permission to relinquish blame and forgive ourselves when something happens that we were unable to predict or avoid. Once Asa was clear on her guideposts, she was able to let go of the missteps that had led to the disconnection with Malik. Rather than nagging him about his grades and punishing him for lying, she focused on his effort and worked on building mutual trust.

Getting the N.A.C. of It

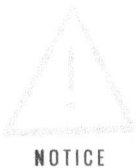

Step 1: NOTICE you need informed decisiveness
Recognize that in every moment you have the power to make a choice. Even when we don't have control over what is happening around us, we still can decide how NOTICE we are going to respond. Simply noticing that we have a choice triggers a reward cue in our brain, which makes us feel more motivated to take action.[65]

---

[65] Association for Psychological Science. "Decisions, decisions, decisions ...." ScienceDaily. ScienceDaily, 19 July 2011. <www.sciencedaily.com/releases/2011/07/110718164207.htm>

Step 2: ASSESS if it's helpful or hurtful

ASSESS

Let's face it, making decisions is risky business because every choice, including not making a choice, comes with consequences. "Good" decisions can have unwelcome or unexpected outcomes; "bad" decisions can end up turning out for the best. There's no way to know for sure what the outcome of our choices will be.

If you're making decisions that go against your guideposts, chances are they're hurtful. When they are aligned with our guideposts, they are helpful. Even when we make a mistake, we can rest assured that we made the best choice we could in the moment.

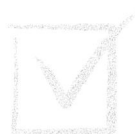

Step 3: CHOOSE what to do next

Choice 1: Stick with it

CHOOSE

You have the choice to continue doing exactly what you've been doing, and you can already predict the outcome. If the outcome is what you want, great. If it's not, just realize that by choosing not to change, there is little chance the outcome will either.

Choice 2: Neutralize it

It's a good idea to postpone making difficult decisions when we're depleted,[66] anxious, or emotionally charged because it narrows our ability to recognize potential solutions.[67] Instead, use a Rapid Reset to

---

[66] Duhigg, Charles. The Power of Habit: Why We Do What We Do in Life and Business. Random House. New York, NY (2012, 2014)

[67] Kounios, J., Frymiare, J.L., Bowden, E.M., Fleck, J.I., Subramaniam, K., Parrish, T.B., & Jung-Beeman, M. (2006). The prepared mind: Neural activity prior to problem presentation predicts solution by sudden insight. Psychological Science, 17, 882-890.

give your brain time to rest so it's energized and able to see things more clearly. This enables us to make far better decisions.[68]

Put your left thumb up (like you're giving a "thumbs up"). Stick out your right pointer finger towards your left thumb. In a simultaneous motion, quickly switch to opposite positions—stick out your left finger at your right thumb. This will take practice, but eventually, you'll train your brain to do it in a swift, seamless motion. This is great to do before starting a task where you need to be laser focused like learning a complex topic, taking a test, playing a game.

Rr   Finger-Thumb Switch

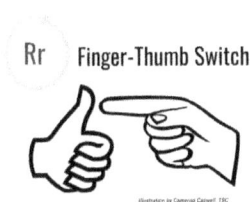

Illustration by Cameron Calwell, TBC

Choice 3: Reframe it

Rather than asking, "What *should* I do?" or "Is this the *right* thing to do?" we can reframe our choices using guideposts. For example, if your guidepost is to be kind, ask, "Is this the kind thing to do?" If your guidepost is to be honest, ask, "Is this the honest thing to do?"

Another tool we can use to make informed decisions is the Path of Possibilities. This simple process can be used by all ages to make decisions of any size or importance.

---

[68] Forte et al., 2021, p. 7

Path of Possibilities

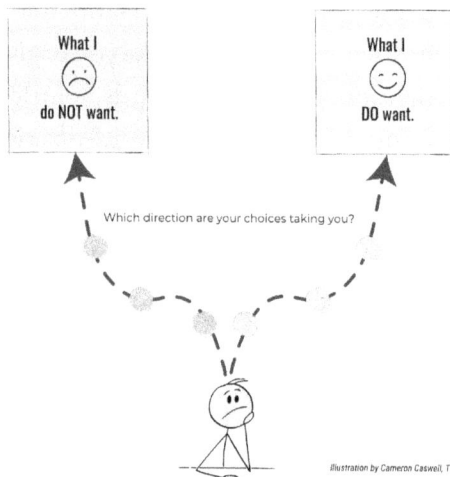

Illustration by Cameron Caswell, TSC

Using the goal of improving relationships with parents as an example, here's how this tool works. First define what you DO want (e.g., *Improve relationships with parents*). Then define what you do NOT want (e.g., *Conflict with parents*). Now consider the decisions you have to make and determine where they fall on the Path of Possibilities (e.g., set up one-on-one meetings or send an accusatory email). Which decisions move you closer to what you DO want and which push you toward what you do NOT want?

Guideposts and the Path of Possibilities also enable us to reframe our bad decisions as unsuccessful decisions. Because we can be confident that we made the best choice based on our guideposts, we're more comfortable accepting accountability for the consequences of our choices. Being accountable, in turn, allows us to learn from our mistakes rather than resorting to excuses and rationalizations. This enables us to continuously improve our proficiency in informed decisiveness.

The Biggest Takeaways

1. When our guideposts are clear and accessible, we are able to make decisions quickly, even effortlessly, that align with WHO we are and what we aspire to DO.
2. Recognize that in every moment you have the power to make a choice.
3. The Path of Possibilities helps us make decisions that move us closer to where we want to go.

CHAPTER 7

~

Social Plasticity

"Well functioning people are able to accept individual differences and acknowledge the humanity of others." [69]

–Dr. Bessel van der Kolk, MD, Author

A re you a Republican or Democrat? Bengals or Pittsburgh fan? Apple or Android user?

Associating with a group not only fulfills our craving to belong, but it also lays a foundation for our identity and self-esteem.[70] It gives us universal guidelines for how to feel, think, and act,[71] especially for those in the midst of trying to figure out who they are (e.g., adolescents). It's a survival instinct. The stronger our connection is to a group, the more secure we feel. Though this seems positive and non-threatening, it is detrimental to those who reside in the out-group.

---

[69] The Body Keeps the Score, van der Kolk, Ch. 5, 17:13-20

[70] https://www.researchgate.net/publication/281208338_Social_Identity_Theory

[71] Brewer, M. B. (1979). In-group bias in the minimal intergroup situation: A cognitive-motivational analysis. Psychological bulletin, 86, 2, 307-324.

The Problem: Judging People Unfairly

Just as we view people within our group more favorably, we tend to view people outside our group as inferior and less desirable. If we don't seek to understand our differences, we form opinions with limited information, perpetuating prejudices and stereotypes we've implicitly picked up on. These assumptions we then reflexively make are unfair. That is where the real danger lives. When we emphasize the differences between groups it can trigger dislike, fear, and hate towards "the others". Prejudice clouds our judgment and decision-making. When left unchecked, it can cause discrimination[72] which further isolates those who are already marginalized or have no identification to a group at all.

Nasty behavior like teasing or bullying manifests in an attempt to increase a group's status at the expense of the "other's" security. Those who stand out more, looking different than most of the group or who do not quite follow the norm, get quickly ostracized.

> "They call me and my friends NPCs at school," one of our young clients told us. Clueless, we asked, "What's an NPC?" "Non-player character." We had to look it up. They 5re the background characters in a video game that add to the overall experience for actual players, but don't have a story of their own. "Why would they call you that?" "To tell us that we don't matter. That brown girls aren't important." "Who calls you this?" "The brown boys."

We all want to feel important, and no one wants to be excluded. This is how some kids dominate the social game while others fade slowly into oblivion. This social isolation has a huge effect on youth mental health because their need to belong is vital to surviving. More

---

[72] Allport, 1954; Dovidio & Gaertner, 2004

than half of all U.S. children have experienced some kind of trauma,[73] which can hinder their ability to cope, trust others, learn, and sustain wellness.[74 75 76] How we treat them impacts their ability to thrive.

Our Brain Tricks Us Into Believing We're Right

Although we've made tremendous strides, disparities still exist in alarming numbers across nearly every facet of our lives including our schools, often in ways so subtle they are difficult to detect.[77 78] Blame it on our amygdala. Imaging research shows that at its core, prejudice is an innate fear response to anyone we deem substantially different from ourselves: from race, to gender, to sports team affiliation. These prejudices are deeply ingrained into our social norms, and we often don't even recognize they exist.

The most tangible way to demonstrate how our brain can trip us up is through optical illusions. Illusions are created when our brain makes assumptions based on what we think we're seeing, but without critical thought.

---

[73] According to the Centers for Disease Control and Prevention (CDC) https://www.cdc.gov/violenceprevention/acestudy/

[74] J. P. Shonkoff and A. S. Garner. Committee on Psychosocial Aspects of Child and Family Health, Committee on Early Childhood, Adoption, and Dependent Care; and Section on Developmental and Behavioral Pediatrics (2012). "The Lifelong Effects of Early Childhood Adversity and Toxic Stress." Available at: http://pediatrics.aappublications.org/content/pediatrics/early/2011/12/21/peds.2011-2663.full.pdf

[75] Mulcahy, 2019

[76] http://www.samhsa.gov/trauma-violence/types

[77] 26 simple charts to show friends and family who aren't convinced racism is still a problem in America. Retrieved at: https://www.businessinsider.com/us-systemic-racism-in-charts-graphs-data-2020-6

[78] Global Gender Gap Report 2022. Retrieved at: https://www.weforum.org/reports/global-gender-gap-report-2022/in-full

Take a look at the Muller-Lyer Illusion: Which line appears to be longer?[79]

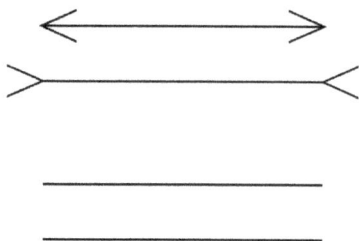

Even when we know that the lines are the same length, we still may struggle to see it because it doesn't jibe with how our brain processes visual cues. And this is straightforward, simple stuff. Imagine how difficult it is for us to wrap our brains around complex cues like behavior, intentions, and emotions.

The problem is that we don't question their accuracy. Once we accept incomplete or distorted information as fact, it's hard to shift out of what we think is true. When we believe we're right, we assume that anyone who sees it differently is wrong.

Let's try it again with the Ebbinghaus Illusion. Which inner circle looks bigger?

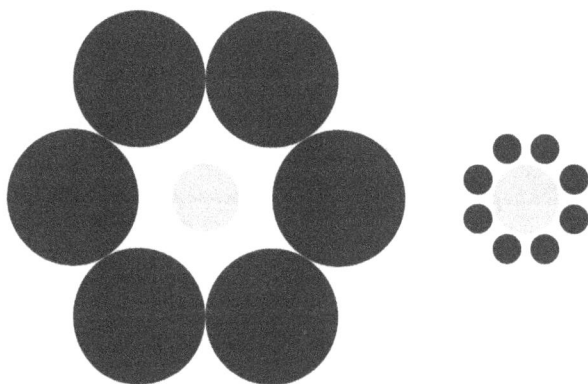

[79] https://www.pnas.org/doi/10.1073/pnas.0409314102

Even now, when we are keenly aware that our brain is tricking us, it's still difficult to process that the inner circles are the same size, isn't it?

Like these visual illusions, we often form a judgment based on our assumptions before we think critically about it. When we don't account for missing or inaccurate information, we're likely to misinterpret what others say and do. We also tend to treat others based on our biased expectations. Because this impacts how they respond to us, it further perpetuates our faulty beliefs.

Why It Matters

This is prevalent in our schools. One out of every five students reports being bullied based on their physical appearance, race/ethnicity, gender, disability, religion, or sexual orientation.[80] Black students, especially boys, and children with learning disabilities are disciplined at alarmingly disproportionate rates.[81] Kids with ADHD get in trouble more when their hyperactivity stands out from other children, doubling their risk of becoming violent by 18 years old.[82] Remember those kids who fell in the river in Chapter 1? These are the ones who were drowning. When we label them, instead of pulling them to safety we send the message that they are not saveable or not good enough to save.

Teachers aren't immune either. We worked with Layla, who told us about an incident she had with her principal:

> I was a new teacher when my principal hauled me into the office and said, "Your expectations of students are too high. Your students are frustrated with you." I became defensive. "Well, I'm

[80] https://www.pacer.org/bullying/info/stats.asp
[81] https://www.gao.gov/assets/gao-18-258.pdf
[82] https://www.ojp.gov/pdffiles1/ojjdp/179065.pdf

frustrated with them!" I said. I was confused. I assumed my principal was being too soft on the kids and too harsh on me. I characterized him as a big jerk. In actuality, his intent was to help me connect with my students, though I didn't understand that until later. He was trying to convey that my students needed me to slow down in my delivery, which I was missing because I was too focused on just getting through the curriculum. If I had asked more questions instead of assuming that he was just trying to assert power over me, I wouldn't have wasted time spinning in anger and could have gained a great mentor instead.

Labels classify WHO they are based on what they DO. Both "good" and "bad" labels negatively distort our perception. We may view one child as a troublemaker and another one as a star pupil. When we pigeonhole people into categories such as sex, race, economic status, and religion, it impacts the way we interact with them. We may continue to mistreat or ignore the troublemaker and lavish attention on the star pupil. This shapes our assumptions and widens differences. It also alters the child's trajectory. When students worry about getting treated unfairly because of their differences, they are more likely to engage in delinquent behavior, like skipping classes, verbally abusing someone, or vandalizing school property.[83] When we're not willing to stop using the distorted lens, harmful stereotypes are perpetuated and the cycle continues.

Conversely, studies show that when educators counter their prejudices and treat these students as though they *will* do well or *can* act better, they do! Sometimes they even excel well beyond their cohorts![84]

---

[83] https://www.gsb.stanford.edu/faculty-research/publications/threats-social-identity-can-trigger-social-deviance

[84] Rosenthal and Jacobson (1968)

Because it's evident this cycle occurs in our schools, although often unintentionally, we have to acknowledge its powerful effect. Protecting kids from further hardship as they move through our school system paves a better life path for them. We want our schools to be safe havens, but when we neglect to reinforce safety it breeds division.

The Current Solution: Inclusion and Equity Programs

Part of what makes teaching a challenging career is the diversity of the students. For the past three decades, we've been trying to remediate the long-standing problem of discrimination by establishing guidelines and mandating training sessions to promote equity and inclusion.

However, research shows that some equity and inclusion programs may create more harm for the groups they are trying to protect and ultimately set inclusion efforts back.[85] [86]

In the podcast series "Nice White Parents,"[87] Chaya Joffe-Walt tells the story of a group of wealthy white families that painfully exacerbated educational inequities in their attempt to minimize it. They came into a school populated mainly by Black, Latino, and Middle Eastern children with the vision of generously giving this poor, diverse group new opportunities. Rather than working with the existing PTA to understand their needs, they barreled ahead to implement a French immersion program. As one of the parents pretentiously explained to the school's principal, "Being bilingual makes a person more sophisticated." Although well-intentioned,

[85] https://hbr.org/2016/07/why-diversity-programs-fail

[86] https://sites.duke.edu/dukeidlab/files/2018/07/WhiteYouthSocialization. pdf

[87] https://podcasts.apple.com/us/podcast/nice-white-parents/id1524080195

they completely missed the mark. The new program made the original group of students feel uncomfortable and unwelcome in their own school.

Why It's Not Solving the Problem

One problem is we're trying to fix deep-seeded, long-term historical issues embedded in societal structures with surface-level, short-term solutions. Another problem is that we are putting the burden on teachers to be more equitable and inclusive, without addressing why these inequities exist in the first place. Many are already trying their best to help students,[88] so simply asking them to do better is adding to the problem, not resolving it. No matter how good our intentions are, without acknowledgment of our implicit biases and their effect on our thoughts and actions, we will stay stuck in the same patterns.

In response to the Truth and Reconciliation Commission of Canada (TRC)[89], Ms. Thompson enthusiastically embraced teaching this rich history in her class. The goal was to educate youth about the generational trauma they endured for decades. She invited indigenous speakers to facilitate cultural activities like smudging and moccasin crafting. She encouraged students to wear orange shirts on September 30th to spread awareness. Ms. Diaz believed she was being a great advocate for the TRC. In one instance, Ms. Diaz asked an indigenous educator a question about smudging and immediately could tell from their reaction it came off offensively. She felt guilty. Later, Ms. Thompson requested another educator to come into her classroom. They explained that the

---

[88] Quaglia & Corso (2016)
[89] https://www.rcaanc-cirnac.gc.ca/eng/1450124405592/1529106060525

activities undermined the sanctity of their culture and removed them from the program. Ms. Thompson scaled back her teaching on the topic altogether because she didn't want to devalue any of the TRC legacy or offend anyone (again). Because educators who had no ties to indigenous communities, like Ms. Diaz, were the ones teaching it, meaningful parts of the story were missing. The program fizzled out.

When we're uncomfortable, we avoid the important conversations necessary to learn and heal. We sit idle. Having these conversations moves us forward. Only when we understand the underlying inequities can we intrinsically change our attitudes and perceptions. This requires safe environments and genuine curiosity from one another. Without inherent change, we may silently endure our differences and learn to control our bias externally[90] in order to avoid judgment or repercussions. Hiding contempt towards others, especially without understanding what it stems from, doesn't make it go away. It may even grow stronger.[91] When we're left to figure it out on our own, we might resort to unhealthy ways of expressing it (violence, abuse). This is also contributing to the stubborn polarization we experience within our school communities today.

The TSC Solution: Social Plasticity

It would be ideal if we could prevent ourselves from making assumptions in the first place, but our brain relies on them to process information quickly. So it's just not going to happen. Instead, we want to rewire our innate response to reflexively seek more information rather than making

---

[90] Plant & Devine, 1998
[91] Greenwald, McGee, & Schwartz, 1998; Olson & Fazio, 2003

a quick judgment. Fortunately, research supports the theory that bias—both explicit and implicit—is amenable to change.[92] In fact, the very belief that we can change is what gives us the capacity to do so.[93]

Social plasticity scrutinizes our own biases and assumptions about people with *curiosity* rather than criticism. It acknowledges that everyone has their own deep, complex narrative which defines and explains WHO they are and what they DO. Because we don't have the full context or access to their inner thoughts and feelings, we accept that we'll never fully understand their perspective. Therefore, we have no recourse for judgment or criticism.

Social Plasticity

PURPOSE: Protect others.
HOW: Curiosity Chain

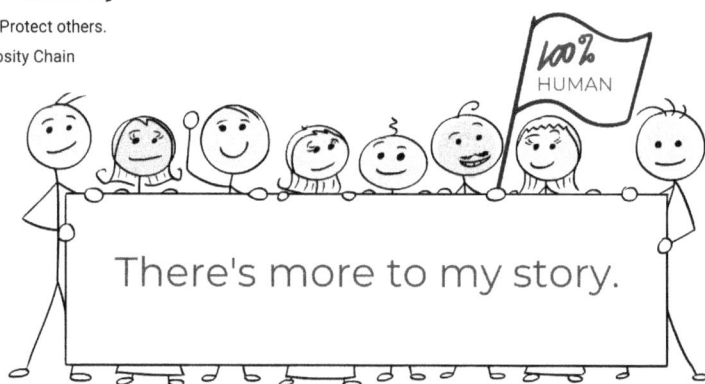

Illustration by Cameron Caswell, TSC with @zdeneksasek via Canva.com

---

[92] Blair, 2002; Kawakami, Dovidio, & van Kamp, 2007; Olson & Fazio, 2006; Page-Gould, Mendoza-Denton, Alegre, & Siy, 2010; Wittenbrink et al., 2001

[93] Carr, P. B., Dweck, C. S., & Pauker, K. (2012, June 18). "Prejudiced" Behavior Without Prejudice? Beliefs About the Malleability of Prejudice Affect Interracial Interactions. Journal of Personality and Social Psychology. Advance online publication. doi: 10.1037/a0028849

The Curiosity Chain

To develop Social Plasticity, we replace our initial snap assumptions with the new assumption, "I don't know the full story." This prompts the simple question, "What am I missing?" We call it the Curiosity Chain.

Curiosity Chain

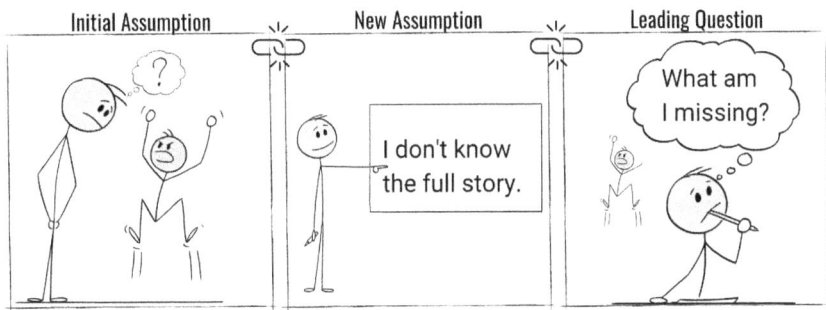

Illustration by Cameron Caswell, TSC with ©zdeneksasek via Canva.com

The Curiosity Chain enables us to seek out more accurate information in order to make a fair assessment. If the parents at the private school had replaced their assumption that the "diverse" children would benefit from learning French and replaced it with the assumption that there was more to their story, they could have discovered that the children were already proficient in Spanish. They may have leveraged that skill to create a more integrated learning experience by teaching the new kids the same language. If Ms. Thompson had replaced the assumption that she offended the indigenous educator with the assumption that there was more to the story, she may have learned that the question she asked made the educator uncomfortable because it reminded him of a past experience and had nothing to do with her. She could have responded with empathy and allowed for the opportunity to explore better solutions rather than dismantling the program altogether.

Using Social Plasticity bridges the social gap and allows us to come together as human beings. It gives us the space to have different opinions, beliefs, or practices without feeling threatened, offended, or upset.

Getting the N.A.C of It

NOTICE

Step 1: NOTICE you need social plasticity
First we must notice that we are making an assumption. It's OK. Everyone does. Remember to notice with curiosity, not criticism.

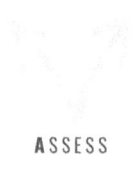

ASSESS

Step 2: ASSESS if it's helpful or hurtful
If you are assuming someone's intention is bad based on a single characteristic (e.g., they have tattoos), a group affiliation (e.g., a particular political party) or label (teenager, ADHD), your assumption could be hurtful. This illusion can prompt us to devalue, dehumanize, even demonize people based on minimal information. This explains why even decent people are able to justify bullying, mistreating, and ostracizing others.

If you are assuming someone's intention is good based on a single characteristic (e.g., they have the same color skin as me) or a group affiliation (e.g., they go to the same church), your assumption could be hurtful. This false sense of security can make even vigilant people susceptible to exploitation, deception, and assault.

Because we naturally resist changing our initial impressions about someone, all invalidated assumptions, both "good" or "bad," risk being hurtful.

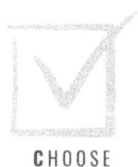

CHOOSE

Step 3: CHOOSE what to do next

Choice #1: Stick with it
You have the choice to continue doing exactly what you've been doing, and you can already predict the outcome. If the outcome is what you want, great. If it's not, just realize that by choosing not to change, there is little chance the outcome will either.

Also, realize that when we get stuck in our judgment we are likely to:

1. Mislabel and misguide others, especially when we're in a position of power.
2. Provoke more internal and external conflict, and possibly do more harm.
3. Close ourselves off from opportunities and solutions.

Choice #2: Neutralize it
It's a good idea to stop ourselves before we make a snap judgment. Instead, use a Rapid Reset to give your brain time to rest so it is better able to see things more critically.

Rr   **Stop Sign**

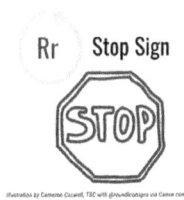

Illustration by Cameron Ciswell, TSC with @roundicongro via Canva.com

Picture a stop sign in your head. Envision yourself tracing the outline of the stop sign and see the word STOP grow from small to large. Continue repeating this process until you no longer feel the urge to take an impulsive action.

Choice #3: Reframe it
Being equitable doesn't mean treating everyone the same; it means giving everyone what they need. Social plasticity helps us consider

each child's unique background, needs, and learning style. We start by replacing our initial assumptions with the assumption, "there is more to the story." Next, ask the leading question, "What am I missing?" Focus on separating WHO the other person is from what they DO. This also prevents us from inaccurately assuming good or bad intentions. If you're struggling to reframe your assumptions, it may be helpful to remember that no matter how different we appear to be on the outside, or how wide apart our beliefs may be, genetically we are 99.99% the same.[94]

The Biggest Takeaways

1. Acknowledge that we all make assumptions and have bias.
2. The Curiosity Chain replaces our initial assumption with the new assumption, "We don't know the full story."
3. All invalidated assumptions, both "good" or "bad," risk being hurtful.

---

[94] https://humanorigins.si.edu/evidence/genetics

CHAPTER 8

~

Empathetic Listening

*"You never really understand a person until you
consider things from his point of view…until you
climb into his skin and walk around in it."*

–Harper Lee, To Kill a Mockingbird

O ne of the most fundamental human needs is a sense of belonging. We are wired to connect with one another. We yearn to be
acknowledged, valued, and heard by those around us at home, in
the classroom, on a team, or in a group. Although we are technically more
"connected" today,[95] [96] we've never felt more alone and disconnected.[97] [98]

The Problem: Social Isolation

Our increasing social engagement doesn't satisfy our need for connection because it confuses feeling lonely with being alone. Although

---

[95] Kahneman et al. (2004)

[96] Kemp (2022)

[97] Cigna (2020)

[98] Murthy (2020)

social media may give us the illusion of being more connected with our friends,[99] it lacks sincerity and gratification.[100] In reality, we could spend the majority of our time surrounded by people and still feel socially isolated. Conversely, we could live relatively solitary lives and not feel lonely. That's because loneliness is based on perceived social isolation, not objective social isolation.

Whether disconnection is real or perceived, it can provoke feelings of anxiety, hurt, anger, even hostility, suspicion, contempt, and aggression.[101] We feel vulnerable and threatened and may start to avoid social interactions to protect ourselves,[102] setting in motion a reinforcing cycle that makes it increasingly more difficult to connect with others.[103]

Currently one in three students does NOT feel like they belong in school[104] and many wish they had more people outside of their family that cared about them or at least asked them how they were doing.[105]

Why It Matters

Dr. Vivek H. Murthy, the 19th Surgeon General of the United States, calls loneliness an epidemic, stating, "During my years caring for patients, the most common condition I saw was not heart disease or

---

[99] https://www.pewresearch.org/internet/2022/08/10/teens-social-media-and-technology-2022/

[100] Bouffard, S., Giglio, D., & Zheng, Z. (2022). Social Media and Romantic Relationship: Excessive Social Media Use Leads to Relationship Conflicts, Negative Outcomes, and Addiction via Mediated Pathways. Social Science Computer Review, 40(6), 1523–1541. https://doi.org/10.1177/08944393211013566

[101] Watson & Nesdale (2012)

[102] Cacioppo (2009)

[103] Newall et al. (2009)

[104] OECD. (2019)

[105] Weissbourd et al. (2021)

diabetes; it was loneliness."[106] Even before the global pandemic, three in five Americans described themselves as lonely.[107] When our need for connection isn't met, it reduces our ability to empathize, trust, and take different perspectives, which are all essential for creating a sense of acceptance and belonging.[108]

The impact of disconnection, perceived rejection, and loneliness is devastating within our school system. It puts kids at risk of using maladaptive coping mechanisms (self-harm, drugs) and leads to higher academic anxiety,[109] anger issues, low self-esteem[110] and eventually, school dropout. This is especially concerning for students who are already vulnerable.[111] Middle schoolers, in particular, are subjected to higher rates of suspensions, detentions, stereotyping, bullying, discrimination, and assault.[112] These negative effects can continue into adulthood.[113]

One teacher reported that at the beginning of his career, he punished students who were "misbehaving" by sending them to other classrooms to isolate them from their peers. As added intimidation, he put them in with students several years older. Although it did deter most students from acting out in the short-term, they were deprived of connection.

Educators also fare negatively when they feel disconnected from their colleagues and school community. They are more prone to absenteeism, low productivity, and quitting.[114] If your students and educators aren't doing well, neither will your school.

---

[106] Murthy (2020)

[107] Cigna (2020)

[108] Konrath et al. (2010)

[109] Gul (2017)

[110] Sandstrom & Zakriski (2004)

[111] Aerts et al. (2012)

[112] Way & Nelson (2018)

[113] Hagerty et al. (2002)

[114] Cigna (2020)

However, when educators feel they belong at a school, they are more engaged, energized, and fulfilled.[115] And when students have positive school-life experiences that increase their sense of belonging, such as positive peer relationships and feeling supported by educators, it can drive their success in the classroom.[116] Teacher support also helps students better cope with difficulties and challenges.

If feeling connected is requisite for students' motivation to learn and feeling valued is essential for educators ability to create strong connections with their students, it would seem that making belongingness a prerogative would be a no brainer. In fact, according to the Organisation for Economic Co-operation and Development (OECD), belonging is a major educational trend for the future.[117]

The Current Solution: Active Listening

One particularly endorsed social skill for making someone feel more connected and valued is listening.[118] Listening–*really* listening–can provide the social support needed to boost a person's self-confidence, build their resilience, earn their trust, inspire a higher level of commitment and motivation, and reduce conflict. There is a benefit to listening to the listener as well. Being a great listener is one of the most effective techniques for increasing our influence and likeability,[119] the most important characteristic of a good leader.[120] On the flip side, poor

---

[115] https://www.qualtrics.com/experience-management/industry/teacher-retention/

[116] Joyce HD. Does school connectedness mediate the relationship between teacher support and depressive symptoms? Child Sch. 2019;41(1):7–16. doi:10.1093/cs/cdy024

[117] https://www.oecd.org/education/trends-shaping-education-22187049.htm

[118] https://www.ncbi.nlm.nih.gov/pmc/articles/PMC8350774/#B52

[119] How to win friends and influence people (1936)

[120] https://www.researchgate.net/publication/319444594_Team_Listening_Environment_TLE

listening can result in turnover, burnout, job dissatisfaction, and low commitment.[121]

Although communication and learning requires us to listen three times more than to read or write, the amount of skills training we receive is in the reverse order.[122] By one account, less than 2% of the population has been formally taught how to listen.[123] That may explain why most of us think we're good listeners but are actually pretty terrible at it.[124] In fact, the average adult listens at only about 25% efficiency.[125]

There are several styles of quality listening that are currently being taught. One of the most well-known is active listening. To listen actively, we must make eye contact, give our undivided attention, use open body language, nod, reflect, paraphrase, ask open-ended questions, and label emotions.[126] The goal of listening actively is to understand what is being said both verbally and nonverbally[127] and to make the person feel heard and respected.

Why It's Not Solving the Problem

One problem we've seen when people attempt active listening, is that they tend to get distracted with the mechanics of it: the way we sit, where we look, when we nod, what words to use (or not use). These are great guidelines to get started, but when we're so focused on what we're doing to appear to be listening, we end up replacing one internal

---

[121] Pery et al., 2020)

[122] Atwater, E., (1992). I hear you. (Rev. ed.). Pacific Grove, Ca.: Walker.

[123] Gregg, G. (1983, September). "They have ears, but hear not": Would a course in listening help? Across the Board, 56-61.

[124] Axley, S., (1996) Communication at work: management and the communication- intensive Organization. Westport, Conn: Quorum

[125] Hunsaker, R. A. (1990). Understanding and developing the skills of oral communication: Speaking and listening (2nd ed.). Englewood, CO

[126] Hybels & Weaver, Communicating Effectively 2015

[127] Nemec, Spagnolo, & Soydon, 2017

dialogue with another. We're still too distracted to give the person our full attention—and they can tell.

Active listening is also challenging if we've already made an assumption, disagree with their perspective, or believe we know what is best for them. We may be tempted to act like we're listening in order to force our own agenda or elicit the response we want. But when we exert our own opinions and judgment into the mix or try to negate how the other person feels, we immediately invalidate them. Telling someone not to feel bad doesn't stop them from feeling bad; in fact, it often makes them feel worse. This includes trying to cheer someone up by saying, "It's not so bad," "Look on the bright side," or "There's no need to feel that way." When we overstate the positive perspective of the situation rather than address the reality of the pain or discomfort it is causing someone, it undermines a person's experience. This phenomenon has been coined "toxic positivity."

Even young kids feel patronized and manipulated by insincere listening. We know we've missed the mark when our attempts at validation are met with a huff of exasperation, eye roll, or "Don't give me that psychobabble" response.

One of our clients, Gabriel, was frustrated because his son, Kai, had a fit every time he asked him to put his video game down. Kai would screech, stomp, threaten to hurt himself—anything he could think of to get out of doing what was asked of him. Gabriel had had enough. He decided to give listening a try. The next time Kai acted up, Gabriel leaned in, looked him in the eye, and calmly said, "You seem angry." Gabriel was expecting this to soothe Kai so that he would feel heard and finally do as he was asked. Instead, Kai became more agitated and yelled louder. What happened? Kai saw right through Gabriel's ploy. Rather than using this strategy to genuinely understand what Kai was feeling, he used it with the intent to get Kai to comply. Because he still didn't understand why Kai was upset, his canned response made Kai feel dismissed.

The TSC Solution: Empathetic Listening

We believe that if people can master a deeper kind of listening in a more genuine, accessible way, we can improve safety, inclusivity, acceptance, and kindness, ultimately nurturing a more positive school culture. This is why we have identified Empathetic Listening as the second essential Allo skill.

Empathetic listening moves beyond the mechanics of active listening attuning to the perspective, emotions, and behaviors of others with genuine empathy. We seek to meet the other person's need to feel valued, heard, and seen.

The key to connecting with someone and making them feel heard and understood is being sincerely curious. Curiosity enhances the path to empathy. We listen with the intent to immerse ourselves fully into their shoes and see through their eyes:

What are they feeling?

Why are they feeling that way?

What is the story they are telling themselves?

Only when we can embrace their perspective will we be able to express true empathy.

Empathetic Listening

PURPOSE: Connect to others.
HOW: Look through their lens.

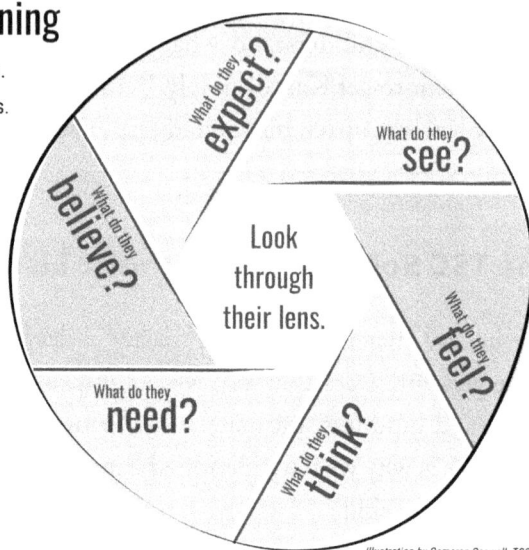

What do they expect?

What do they see?

What do they believe?

Look through their lens.

What do they feel?

What do they need?

What do they think?

Illustration by Cameron Caswell, TSC

Because we genuinely focus on trying to see the situation through their eyes, the mechanics naturally fall into place. When we pay attention to all the ways they communicate what they are experiencing, we automatically tune out the environment and get laser-focused on them. When we are able to find similarities between their experience and our own, it becomes easier to give a heartfelt response.

If Gabriel had used empathetic listening he would have asked questions like, "What's it like to play video games?", "Why is playing video games so important to you?", and "What are you thinking when I ask you to stop?" Using questions like this, Gabriel would have learned that Kai was struggling with severe anxiety and playing video games was the only thing that gave him relief. By knowing this, Gabriel could have changed his approach by letting go of his inaccurate assumptions and expectations and worked with Kai to find a solution that addressed his needs.

Listening empathically also requires us to release our need to be right and control the situation. When we acknowledge that what another person feels is non-negotiable, we no longer feel the need to impose what we think they should be feeling or thinking. Only then can we truly validate them and make them feel valuable and significant. This is how we increase social connectedness and reduce loneliness.[128]

Listening with empathy also energizes us and elevates those around us. Once it becomes an automated response, we are able to have more meaningful exchanges within a shorter period of time. Empathetic listening is also contagious.[129] People who are shown empathy, are likely to pay it forward by showing empathy to the next person.[130] All it takes is a handful of people genuinely listening to each other to set off a wave of kindness and compassion. It could be a teacher noticing a student is out of sorts and asking what they can do to help. Or an administrator checking in with a teacher to make sure they have what they need to do their job well. Wouldn't that be a wonderful space to be in?

Lena, a paraeducator we worked with, changed her strategy after learning empathetic listening. She was getting frustrated with one of her senior students, Eli, who missed a lot of classes. Persistent calls home weren't motivating him to get there more regularly; it only caused more tension. When Lena listened to Eli to find out the underlying reason--that he only needed to pass the class to graduate--she was able to validate why the class was a low priority to him. Now they were able to work out a plan for the rest of the semester.

---

[128] https://jamanetwork.com/journals/jamapsychiatry/fullarticle/2765959

[129] https://ethicsunwrapped.utexas.edu/glossary/prosocial-behavior

[130] Christakis, N. A., & Fowler, J. H. (2013). Social contagion theory: examining dynamic social networks and human behavior. Statistics in medicine, 32(4), 556–577. https://doi.org/10.1002/sim.5408

When this skill is used consistently and proficiently, it will reduce frustration and conflict and educators can spend more time creating learning experiences rather than managing disruptive behaviors. Now that's something worth listening to!

Getting the N.A.C. of It

NOTICE

Step 1: NOTICE you need empathetic listening
All humans need to be heard. So at any moment there is an opportunity for you to listen with empathy. Notice how you are responding to those opportunities. Sometimes we want to listen, but we can't or we won't for various reasons. We might have to use the bathroom, head to an important meeting, or tend to someone else in need. We get that. Perhaps it's just not the right time. Remember to notice with curiosity, not criticism.

ASSESS

Step 2: ASSESS if it's helpful or hurtful
The extent to which we make the person we're listening to feel validated is a strong indicator of whether we're being helpful or hurtful. You can tell if someone feels validated or not by their response. If they become more open, relaxed, and trusting, you're on the right track. If they start to shut down, get agitated, or suspicious, you're probably not.

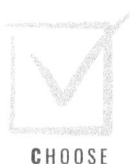

CHOOSE

Step 3: CHOOSE what to do next

Choice #1: Stick with it
You have the choice to continue doing exactly what you've been doing, and you can already predict the outcome. If the outcome is what you want, great. If it's not, just realize that by choosing not to change, there is little chance the outcome will either.

Choice #2: Neutralize it

If the person you're trying to listen to is communicating in a way that causes you distress or anger, it may be difficult to refrain from judging, commenting, scowling, or retaliating. This is the ideal time to use a Rapid Reset in order to remain calm and collected. The goal isn't to change their mood, but to not let their mood impact yours as you listen with empathy.

Here's a Rapid Reset you can use. Take one deep breath in through your nose as slowly as you can. Now exhale through your mouth as slowly as you can. Repeat until you feel calm.

Rr   Inhale/Exhale

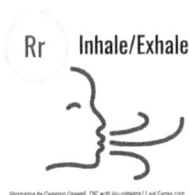

Illustration by Cameron Caswell, TSC with @cumberbily11 via Canva.com

Choice #3: Reframe it

The good news is, we don't have to agree to validate. Instead, listen with the intent to make sense of what they are saying within their current life context or situation–not your own.[131] What thoughts, emotions, and actions are creating the lens through which they are experiencing the world (their story spiral)? Try to see the world through that same lens.

---

[131] Rathus + Miller, 2015, p.54; Linehan, 1993a, pg. 222-223

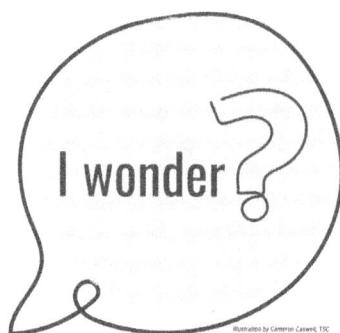

You can start by thinking, "I wonder…" then listen for the answer.

+ I wonder why they feel the need to swear.
+ I wonder why they keep coming to class late.
+ I wonder why they don't hand their homework in on time.
+ I wonder why I get so upset when they question me.

If we can't relate, we can try recalling a personal experience that is either very similar or has a similar theme (e.g., anxiety, embarrassment, frustration, rejection.) Let's say a student is upset because of the amount of homework they have. We may think that they are blowing the situation out of proportion. However, there may have been a time or two that we felt like we had to take on more than our share of responsibilities at home or had to complete a project in a ridiculous amount of time. We may have felt overwhelmed, irritated, mistreated, powerless. When you felt that way, what did you want from other people? Criticism or empathy? Advice or validation?

The Biggest Takeaways

1. All it takes is a handful of people genuinely listening to each other to set off a wave of kindness and compassion.

2. The key to connecting with someone and making them feel heard and understood is being sincerely curious.
3. All humans need to be heard. So at any moment there is an opportunity for you to listen with empathy.

CHAPTER 9

~

Informed
Responsiveness

"Be kind whenever possible. It is always possible."

–Dalai Lama

There has been a significant uptick in disruptive and violent behavior in schools across the country.[132] Because educators now have to spend a "great deal of time and energy to manage the classroom," due to this "intolerable" and "stress-provoking" behavior,[133] school is becoming less about educating students and more about trying to discipline and control them.[134] [135] The responsibility this puts on educators is more than many can handle. Although many educators say that they do not feel equipped or confident enough to respond effectively (as discussed in Chapter 2), the majority report having extraordinary pressure placed on them to address student behavior problems

[132] https://www.edweek.org/leadership/threats-of-student-violence-and-misbehavior-are-rising-many-school-leaders-report/2022/01

[133] https://www.hindawi.com/journals/tswj/2012/208907/

[134] http://www.childhealthdata.org/browse/survey/results

[135] Nakpodia, (2010), Alemayehu (2012) and Oluremi (2013)

themselves. Veteran educators acknowledge this skill gap identifying "poor classroom management" as the top problem among educators.[136]

The Problem: We're Focusing on Behavior

We seem to believe that if we can control kids' behavior, everything would be better. The problem is, we're trying to control the wrong thing. Traditional discipline methodologies are based on the theory that all behavior is simply a response to environmental stimuli and can be re-conditioned through positive and negative reinforcement. Put simply, actions that are rewarded will be repeated and those that are punished will not. This was famously demonstrated by Pavlov's dogs,[137] poor Little Albert,[138] and Skinner's dancing pigeons.[139]

Based on this theory, it seems logical to implement punitive strategies to curb undesirable behavior. This includes harsh verbal reprimands and yelling, physical warnings such as posturing over a student, consequences like taking away free-time or devices, suspension, expulsion, and even corporal punishment.[140] [141] The more painful we make it, the less likely they will repeat it, right?

> One of our clients, Melissa, was fed up with her son's laziness and apathy towards schoolwork. Every day she nagged and yelled at him to get off his video games and get his work done. He would

---

[136] https://tntp.org/assets/documents/TNTP_Perspectives_2013.pdf

[137] Pavlov (1897/1902)

[138] Watson (1920)

[139] Skinner, B. F. (1948). Superstition' in the pigeon. Journal of Experimental Psychology, 38, 168-172.

[140] https://apps.nasponline.org/resources-and-publications/books-and-products/samples/HCHS3_Samples/S4H18_Discipline.pdf

[141] https://www.newsnationnow.com/us-news/education/missouri-school-district-brings-back-spanking/

either ignore her or yell back. She tried removing social distractions by taking his phone away, forbidding him to hang out with his friends, and banning him from playing video games until he "did better." Her son still didn't do his homework, but he did get more belligerent. She couldn't understand why he was making it so difficult for both of them.

Why do we think that doing more of what hasn't worked, is going to work? Even if punishments are successful at curbing immediate behavior, they fail to spark intrinsic motivation and prompt long-term change. That's because we can't control how they feel, what they think, or how they react. When we focus strictly on external behavior and fail to address *why* the behavior exists, it is likely to reoccur or manifest in another maladaptive way. We end up in a loop of whack a mole suppressing a behavior in one place only for it to pop up again somewhere else because they still may be relying on that behavior to get a need met. This approach also assumes that they are capable of changing their behavior and are simply choosing not to.

There are decades of research showing that reactive, punitive responses are not only ineffective, but they also put us at risk of substantial harm which far outweighs any potential benefits. Rather than promoting long-term change, what this does is teach children to temporarily suppress undesirable behavior until the threat of punishment is gone (or they learn to better hide it from the punisher). On the flip side, children (and, let's face it, adults, too) may display desirable behavior in order to obtain a reward, but are less likely to do it once the reward is removed.

The corresponding feelings and needs, which are amplified when they feel manipulated or controlled, are often released through aggression towards others, themselves, or both. Children who refuse to suppress their thoughts, behaviors, and emotions or are unable to do so are often labeled as difficult, defiant, and troubled. Rather than changing to a more effective approach, we bribe them with more rewards or pile on more punishments, which may not be directly related or proportional to the "crime".

When we attempt to coerce or push them to action, we provoke an equally negative reaction instead. The more we try to control, the more out of control our students become.[142]

Logan, a 12th grader, did not return to class after signing out to go to the bathroom. His teacher called down to the office to notify them. The principal checked the cameras and spotted Logan roaming the halls, nowhere near where he was supposed to be. She watched as a staff member, Mr. Young approached Logan and appeared to motion him to go. Logan appeared combative. The principal witnessed Mr. Young getting more agitated and yelling at Logan. As the situation escalated, the school resource officer (SRO) intervened, and Logan was eventually led out of the building in handcuffs.

In a battle of wills, situations can quickly spin out of control. However, when we do nothing and let them "walk all over us," we send the message that the behavior is acceptable or that we don't have the authority to address it. The longer inappropriate behavior continues, the more difficult it is to stop.

---

[142] Cardiff University. "Teenagers less likely to respond to mothers with controlling tone of voice: New study showed adolescents were less likely to want to engage with schoolwork when mothers spoke with a pressurizing tone." Science-Daily. ScienceDaily, 26 September 2019. <www.sciencedaily.com/releases/2019/09/190926202307.htm>.

Mr. Robinson, a 4th grade teacher, was irritated with his new student, Tori, when she refused to do her work during class. She bothered other students by making loud noises, and he had to give frequent prompts like, "Tori, pay attention" or "Tori, stay on task." Tori let out big sighs and seemed agitated in response, often stomping her feet and rolling her eyes. Mr. Robinson was spending so much time focusing on Tori's behavior, the other students weren't getting what they needed. He tried to ignore Tori's disruptive behavior hoping the lack of attention would make it go away. It didn't. One day when Mr. Robinson reminded Tori to start her work, she threw her pencil at him in protest. This is not what he signed up for!

Why It Matters

For decades, experts have been asserting that discipline problems are related more to how adults handle problems than to actual student misconduct.[143] The more we ignore the child's behavior, the more insignificant they feel. The more we assert our power, the more the student feels threatened and unsafe.[144] Additionally, heightened displays of negative emotion towards a child puts them at risk of unnecessary embarrassment and humiliation. Multiply that if done in public. In either extreme, they will instinctively protect themselves with retaliation, resentment, and overall distrust in authority figures.[145] Eventually, most of them shut down altogether,[146] and we've lost them.

---

[143] Duke, D. L. (1978) Adults can be discipline problems too! Psychology in the Schools, 15(4), 522-528

[144] http://www.childhealthdata.org/browse/survey/results

[145] https://docs.google.com/document/d/18D1LUhl-Xnt1kATu55U6sACaX q2vf5FSv6RkX-OAxaM/edi

[146] The Body Keeps the Score, van der Kolk, ch 5 33:15

Even the use of less obvious punitive strategies such as humiliation, fear, and intimidation can hurt a student's long-term well-being and cause them to develop addictions, compulsions, and anxiety.[147] Responses such as reprimanding, criticizing, and restrictions also lower their motivation, impair academic achievement, decrease their willingness to comply with instruction,[148] and threaten their future success.[149]

If Melissa had understood this, she would have realized that her approach was demotivating her son and compounding his stress, rather than setting him up to be happy and successful.

Misinformed reactions can have a ripple effect that extends far beyond the misbehaving child. If a teacher lacks the skills to effectively manage behaviors it creates an unsafe, unpredictable, stressful environment that evokes even more problem behaviors.[150] When educators are stretched thin, they do not have the patience needed to manage behavior effectively.[151][152] In turn, student misbehavior is one of the most significant sources of teacher stress. When educators are consumed with dealing with disruptive behaviors, little time is left for teaching. The

[147] Sava, F. A (2001): Causes and effects of teacher conflict-inducing attitudes towards pupils: A path analysis model. Journal of teaching and teacher education, 18, 1007-1021. https://www.sciencedirect.com/science/article/abs/pii/S0742051X02000562

[148] https://www.ncbi.nlm.nih.gov/pmc/articles/PMC6176062/

[149] Sava, F. A (2001): Causes and effects of teacher conflict-inducing attitudes towards pupils: A path analysis model. Journal of teaching and teacher education, 18, 1007-1021. https://www.sciencedirect.com/science/article/abs/pii/S0742051X02000562

[150] Jennings, P. A., & Greenberg, M. T. (2009)

[151] Ingersoll, R. M. (2001)

[152] Teacher turnover and teacher shortages: An organizational analysis. American Educational Research Journal, 38(3), 499–534; McCormick, J., & Barnett, K. (2011)

learning environment erodes, the quality of education suffers,[153] [154] student academic performance declines, and misbehavior intensifies.[155] [156]

As discussed in Chapter 3, this stress spillover disrupts family life, too. Child misbehavior causes parents to stress and high levels of parenting stress has been associated with impatient, harsh, and negative parenting, which leads to more child misbehavior.[157]

The longer these cycles continue in both school and at home without an effective solution, the worse the problem becomes. Despite gaping holes in logic and decades of evidence that show its ineffectiveness, educators, parents, and schools still depend heavily on using external motivators to modify behavior. But what do we do instead?

The Current Solution: Reparation and Restoration

Many schools are replacing their punitive measures with a restorative approach in response to the growing realization that the zero-tolerance policies of the 1980s and 1990s not only do more harm than good, but are negatively biased toward marginalized and vulnerable students.[158]

Unlike punitive approaches which rely on deterrence to manage behavior and prevent misconduct, restoration focuses on building,

---

[153] Jackl, 2006

[154] Myers, Milne, Baker, & Ginsburg, (1987) https://www.iiste.org/Journals/index.php/JEP/article/viewFile/55118/56930

[155] Myers, Milne, Baker, & Ginsburg, 1987

[156] Baker, Jean & Clark, Teresa & Crowl, Alicia & Carlson, John. (2009). The Influence of Authoritative Teaching on Children's School Adjustment Are Children with Behavioural Problems Differentially Affected?. School Psychology International. 30. 374-382. 10.1177/0143034309106945

[157] Deater-Deckard and Scarr, 1996

[158] Losen, D. (Ed.). (2014). Closing the school discipline gap: Equitable remedies for excessive exclusion. New York, NY: educators College Press

nurturing, and repairing relationships.[159] This approach has been demonstrated to be the most effective way to improve student behavior.[160] It is also strongly linked to better academic scores.[161] By addressing the root causes of behavior issues, teaching and strengthening self-management skills, and repairing relationships between students and staff, this approach is believed to be a more viable solution for improving school culture and keeping students in school.[162] Although this approach has been shown to be highly effective, it needs to be implemented correctly and integrated with other solutions if we're going to solve the mental health crises.

Why It's Not Solving the Problem

Although many schools that implement these strategies have reported significant drops in violent acts and serious incidents,[163] absenteeism,[164][165]

[159] Morrison, B., & Vaandering, D. (2012). Restorative justice: Pedagogy, praxis, and discipline. Journal of School Violence, 11(2), 138–155.

[160] https://journals.sagepub.com/doi/10.1177/1053451208328831

[161] http://bottemabeutel.com/wp-content/uploads/2014/01/Simonson-et-al.-evidence-based-practices.pdf

[162] https://files.eric.ed.gov/fulltext/ED595733.pdf

[163] Lewis, S. (2009). Improving school climate: Findings from schools implementing restorative practices. Bethlehem, PA: International Institute for Restorative Practices.

[164] McMorris, B. J., Beckman, K. J., Shea, G., Baumgartner, J., & Eggert, R. C. (2013). Applying restorative justice practices to Minneapolis Public Schools students recommended for possible expulsion. Minneapolis: University of Minnesota

[165] Jain, S., Bassey, H., Brown, M., & Kalra, P. (2014). Restorative justice in Oakland schools: Implementation and impacts (prepared for the Office of Civil Rights, U.S. Department of Education). Oakland, CA: Oakland Unified School District, Data In Action.

and tardiness,[166] other schools have experienced just the opposite.[167] We uncovered two big reasons why this is.

First, although there is extraordinary value in positive reinforcement and restorative practices, when we approach them as a separate skill or process, it causes inconsistencies. Anytime there is inconsistent implementation and some aspect is applied to one and not the other, it leads to student dissatisfaction and a sense of injustice. When students feel they are treated unfairly, they respond by acting out.[168] Teachers take the brunt of the fall out. They complain that they feel like they have no recourse to address misbehavior and that students take advantage of what they perceive as a lack of consequences.[169] In a New York Post article, one frustrated teacher lamented, "We have educators getting kicked at, spit at, cursed at, things thrown at [them] and the kid is back the next day like nothing happened." They even go as far as blaming the teacher for triggering the child.[170] When these strategies fail to deliver, many schools backslide to more reactive, punitive forms of discipline[171] in an attempt to regain control and safety. These measures then erode the very culture they are trying to build.

The second problem is that these programs may require educators to take on even more responsibilities including training, additional

---

[166] Baker, M. (2009). DPS Restorative Justice Project: Year three. Denver, CO: Denver Public Schools

[167] Riestenberg, N. (2003). Restorative schools grants final report, January 2002–June 2003: A summary of the grantees' evaluation. Roseville, MN: Minnesota Department of Education

[168] Tattum, D. (1982) Disruptive pupils in schools and units (Chichester, John Wiley & Sons).

[169] https://nypost.com/2022/06/04/educators-parents-want-discipline-as-nyc-student-suspensions-fall/

[170] https://nypost.com/2022/06/04/educators-parents-want-discipline-as-nyc-student-suspensions-fall/

[171] https://thenevadaindependent.com/article/finger-pointing-over-school-violence-targets-restorative-justice-law

lessons and instruction, and spending more one-on-one time with students—and do it within the limited hours of the school day. On top of that, the pressure and expectations from leadership to do the "right thing," regardless of their ability, creates more anxiety and depletes educators of the very energy they need to do the "right thing." How can we expect educators and parents to show up for children the way they need to when they have nothing left to give?

The TSC Solution: Informed Responsiveness

How we respond to others impacts the outcome and can be the difference between a situation escalating or being resolved. We know that neither you nor your student is going to be able to respond rationally if you are both being reactive. Unfortunately, even if we have the best intentions to be "chill," it's difficult when a child is refusing to follow instructions, exploding in fits of rage, or being swept away in waves of anxiety. The good news is that emotional reactivity is a learned behavior. That means we can reprogram our reactions by learning to override our primitive emotional brain and re-engage our evolved thinking brain. We do this with Informed Responsiveness.

Think of your emotional response as a ladder. Every time our response does not resolve a problem we move up a rung, for example from irritation to agitation. The higher we climb up the ladder, the more difficult it is to think critically and the further we get from a satisfactory resolution. The real power lies in our ability to avoid getting on the Ladder of Conflict in the first place.

Ladder of Conflict

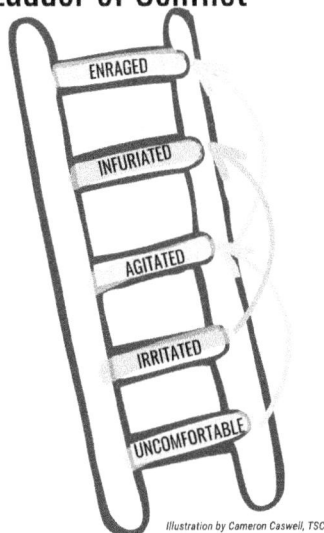

ENRAGED

INFURIATED

AGITATED

IRRITATED

UNCOMFORTABLE

Illustration by Cameron Caswell, TSC

To do this we must parse out what actions and reactions we have control of in the situation, and which we do not. This empowers us to take responsibility for our part and prevents us from being influenced or manipulated by what others think, feel, and do.

Circle of Control

The Circle of Control helps us identify what we actually can impact and, more importantly, what we cannot. Willing others to change may feel like we're taking control of the situation, but it's an illusion. Sure, we can demand that a student sit down and be quiet. They may even do it. But we have no control over how they do it, what they're thinking about it, or how it makes them feel.

The Circle of Control also enables us to change our focus from what they are doing to make us feel a certain way to what assumptions we are making about them that are sparking those emotions. If we feel anxious, frustrated, angry, or resentful it's because we are trying to control something that is not ours to control.

Informed Responsiveness

PURPOSE: Resolve for others.
HOW: Circle of Control.

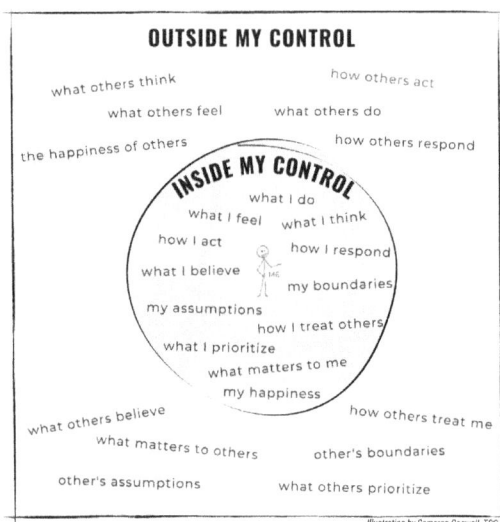

OUTSIDE MY CONTROL

what others think   how others act
what others feel   what others do
the happiness of others   how others respond

INSIDE MY CONTROL
what I do
what I feel   what I think
how I act   how I respond
what I believe
my boundaries
my assumptions
how I treat others
what I prioritize
what matters to me
my happiness

what others believe   how others treat me
what matters to others   other's boundaries
other's assumptions   what others prioritize

Illustration by Cameron Caswell, TSC

Let's go back to Mr. Young and Logan. Most of that story, from the yelling to the handcuffs, could have been prevented had Mr. Young focused on what he could control (e.g., his temper, his words, his tone, his assumptions) rather than trying to control Logan (e.g., his emotions, his response, his words). If he was focused on only his part of the dynamic, he wouldn't have got upset when Logan refused to comply.

When things are within our Circle of Control, we have access to the context behind them. We can tap into our emotions and thoughts. We know what our experiences have been that led us to this moment. When things are outside our Circle of Control, we have minimal to no context. And without context, nothing makes sense. For example, misbehavior may be a child's best defense mechanism or coping strategy. Although it may not serve them well in the moment, in a different context or at another point in time, these behaviors may have served them well and even protected them from harm.

These factors are not excuses for poor behavior, however when we account for them, we can respond more appropriately. For example, if Mr. Young had stepped off the conflict ladder and given Logan some space to calm down, he may have been able to resolve the situation without getting the police involved.

By relinquishing responsibility for what others do, we no longer feel the need to control them.

Getting the N.A.C. of It

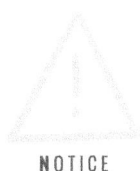

Step 1: NOTICE you need informed responsiveness

NOTICE

Before we can replace a reaction with an informed response, we must first notice when we're reacting. Become familiar with how your stress response shows up in your body and thoughts. What is your default reaction? Do you get defensive? Aggressive? Sensitive? Submissive? Fearful? Do you think, "What's wrong with this person?" or "I need to put a stop to this immediately?!!" Remember to notice with curiosity, not criticism. It may help to remind yourself that your initial feeling is an automatic stress response, not the most effective or logical response.

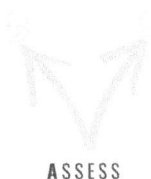

Step 2: ASSESS if it's Helpful or Hurtful

ASSESS

When we respond by further isolating students (e.g., suspensions) or harshly disciplining someone, we can do more harm than good. We can tell if our response is hurtful by noticing the reaction it elicits. If your response exacerbates the behavior of the person you're responding to—they yell louder, cry harder, try to shrink themselves smaller—your response is likely hurtful.

A good litmus test to determine if it's a hurtful response is to ask yourself: "How would I feel if this interaction became a viral video on social media?" If we don't want it to go viral, we may want to rethink our response. Remember, even if it doesn't spread to the masses, our words and actions can impact the other person's sense of safety and feeling of belongingness like a virus.

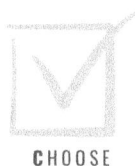

Step 3: CHOOSE what to do next

CHOOSE

Once you notice that split second between a trigger event and your knee-jerk reaction, hit the "pause" button. You now can make an informed decision about what to do next.

Choice #1: Stick with it

You have the choice to continue doing exactly what you've been doing, and you can already predict the outcome. If the outcome is what you want, great. If it's not, just realize that by choosing not to change, there is little chance the outcome will either.

Choice #2: Neutralize it

Rr   Ladder of Conflict

Illustration by Cameron Crowell, TSC

When you're aware that you are feeling discomfort, picture yourself freezing on the bottom rung of the ladder, and slowly climb down. If you've already climbed up, it's OK. Picture yourself freezing there and slowly climbing back down. This visual reminder will help alter your physical and emotional state, bringing you back to *calm*.

Choice #3 Reframe it

Let's revisit the story of Mr. Robinson and Tori for an example of reframing using our Circle of Control. When we left them earlier in the chapter, Tori had just thrown her pencil at Mr. Robinson, and he was getting frustrated. He thought, "What is inside my Circle of Control?"

Mr. Robinson ended up calling Tori's mom (inside his Circle of Control) and found out that Tori was in the midst of trying a new medication for a recently diagnosed illness. This particular medicine sometimes caused agitation. Since Tori had concentration issues inherently on top of this, she had difficulty maintaining her cool throughout the long school day. Tori's mom shared a few tricks that helped her remain calm and on task in the following days.

The Biggest Takeaways

1. The higher we climb up the Ladder of Conflict, the more difficult it is to come to a resolution.
2. The Circle of Control helps us identify what we actually can impact and, more importantly, what we cannot.
3. A good litmus test to determine if our response is hurtful is to ask: "How would I feel if this interaction became a viral video on social media?"

CHAPTER 10

∽

Relationship
Reciprocity

*"I can be changed by what happens to me.
But I refuse to be reduced by it."*

–Maya Angelou

Our relationships are as critical to our survival and well-being as food, water, and shelter. They are the single biggest predictor of our happiness—even more so than business success, physical health, wealth, or status. [172] Relationships provide us with protection, help, support, and acceptance. That only works, however, when both parties have a positive emotional experience. [173] [174]

---

[172] Harvard Study of Adult Development. Retrieved at: https://www.adult-developmentstudy.org

[173] Lim, M., Allen, K. A., Craig, H., Smith, D., & Furlong, M. (2021). Feeling lonely and a need to belong: What is shared and distinct? Australian Journal of Psychology. https://doi.org/10.1080/00049530.2021.1883411.

[174] Hawkins, J. D., & Weis, J. G. (1985). The social development model: An integrated approach to delinquency prevention. Journal of Primary Prevention, 6(2), 73–97.

The Problem: Imbalance of Power

Trust and respect are foundational to every healthy, gratifying relationship. They are also two of the most difficult qualities to build and sustain. This is because we all expect others to respect and trust us, but we're often resistant to trust and respect others. They both require us to be vulnerable, which are associated frequently with being weak. It opens us up to possible pain, humiliation, and regret. No one wants that.

If everyone expects to get trust and respect, but few want to give trust and respect, our expectations are often left unmet. Unmet expectations create dissatisfaction and resentment. It also creates a perceived or real imbalance of power. Rarely, do we feel like that imbalance is in our favor.

Giving too much

> While driving her son, Liam, to practice, Cicely asked him a question about his homework. Liam didn't reply. She glanced over and noticed that he had his earbuds in and hadn't heard her. She tapped him on the shoulder and motioned for him to take the ear buds out. Liam scowled and snapped, "Why?! Can't you see I'm listening to something!" Cicely was furious. In her head she seethed, "I feed him, I put a roof over his head, I drive him to the ends of the earth and back, not to mention I spent eight hours in labor giving birth to him. The least he could do is show me a smidgen of respect."

When we give in a relationship, we expect to get the same amount in return, or at least somewhere in the same ballfield. This includes getting adequate appreciation for what we give. When we don't, we perceive it as the other person letting us down. We may feel disrespected, ignored, even abused. We get angry. We feel hurt. When we feel our happiness is dependent on what others do, it creates the illusion that they have power over us.

- We provide our kids with everything they could possibly need and more. We expect them to be grateful. When they fail to even say thank you or worse, complain, we get angry at them for taking us for granted.
- We spend hours preparing amazing learning experiences for our students. We expect them to pay attention. When they disrupt the class, we resent them for disrespecting us.
- We listen to our friend go on and on about their personal drama. We expect them to listen to our drama, too. When they leave without even asking how we're doing, we get angry for being a doormat.

Taking too much

In some relationships the imbalance of power is more extreme. This is especially true when there is a person with more authority. People often misconstrue authority as having the right to respect and trust. If others don't give it to them willingly, they may feel justified in using control or manipulation to take it:

- Parents may punish their children for lying to them and demand that they tell them the truth. In other words, they try to force them to give them trust.
- Educators may reprimand students for being rude and humiliate them in front of their classmates until they apologize. In other words, force them to give them respect.

Control and manipulation may also show up in more subtle, yet equally damaging ways. This could be threatening with consequences, belittling and insulting, and undermining or invalidating feelings and experiences. Whatever form it takes, unhealthy control usually revolves around limiting a person's autonomy and blaming them for causing our negative emotions.

> Cicely's irritation continued to grow during the drive. When she couldn't stand it any longer, she leaned over and snatched one of the ear buds out of Liam's ear and yelled, "You listen to me when I'm talking to you. Don't you ever disrespect me like that again." Liam rolled his eyes, grabbed the ear bud back from Cicely, and put it back in his ear. That was more than Cicely could tolerate. She swerved the car to the side of the road, put it into park, and screeched, "I'm done with you. Either take those earbuds out RIGHT NOW or you can get out and walk the rest of the way. Either way, you're not getting those earbuds back until you learn to respect me. I'm sick of you upsetting me."

Expecting too much

Although these tactics may eventually result in compliant behavior, the appearance of trust and respect is superficial. Genuine trust and respect cannot be demanded. In fact, the very act of demanding them is likely to diminish them instead.

> During his therapy session the next day, Liam ranted about his mom. He was tired of her telling him what he should do and how he should act. No matter how hard he tried, she just found something else to yell at him about. He couldn't do anything right. He

> was counting down the days until he could finally move out and be free of her.

When we blame the other person for our unmet expectations, we send the message that, "If you were a good person, you would do this, but you're not doing it; therefore:

+ YOU are not enough.
+ YOU are a disappointment.
+ I don't trust YOU.
+ YOU are a failure.
+ YOU should be ashamed.
+ My love for YOU is conditional."

Chances are this is NOT what the other person was expecting from you. Now they feel let down by you and by themselves.

When we feel mistreated or disappointed, we may hide behind defense mechanisms like anger, attitude, and isolation. Other times, we try harder. We see clients who are in a constant state of anxiety trying to predict what is expected of them. They feel like they're constantly walking on eggshells to avoid setting someone off. They're laden with guilt and shame when they aren't successful.

Why It Matters

When there is an unhealthy imbalance of power, either real or perceived, we start to view each other through a lens of contempt, resentment, and fear. Rather than finding refuge in the relationship, we feel unsafe, even victimized. This can lead to lower self-esteem, perceptions of social support, and hope for the future, which puts our mental health at risk. [175]

Poor relationships between students and educators has been identified as one of the biggest impediments to developing social and communication skills.[176] Likewise, children with parents who are overly controlling tend to have lower moral reasoning, self-regulation, social skills, and academic success.[177] In contrast, when students are treated with respect and feel supported by their educators and parents, they tend to be more academically successful and well-adjusted.[178] Similarly, positive relationships reduce teacher and staff burnout and improve their well-being, motivation, and satisfaction with work.[179] Because they play such an important role in our emotional fitness, the U.S. Army actively teaches its soldiers how to build solid relationships.[180] How powerful would it be if more students, educators, and parents had these skills as well?

---

[175] Mays, V. M., & Cochran, S. D. (2001). Mental health correlates of perceived discrimination among lesbian, gay, and bisexual adults in the United States. American Journal of Public Health, 91, 1869–1876. http://dx.doi.org/10.2105/AJPH.91.11.1869). https://www.apa.org/pubs/journals/releases/spq-spq0000373.pdf

[176] Neidell, M., & Waldfogel, J. (2010). Cognitive and noncognitive peer effects in early education. The Review of Economics and Statistics, 92, 562–576. http://dx.doi.org/10.1162/REST_a_00012

[177] Baumrind D. 1966. Effects of authoritative parental control on child behavior. Child Development, 37(4), 887-907.

[178] Kim, J. (2021). The quality of social relationships in schools and adult health: Differential effects of student–student versus student–teacher relationships. School Psychology, 36(1), 6–16. https://doi.org/10.1037/spq0000373

[179] Krieger, L. & Sheldon, K. (2015) What MakesLawyers Happy? A Data-Driven Prescription to Redefine Professional Success retrieved at: https://ir.law.fsu.edu/cgi/viewcontent.cgi?article=1093&context=articles

[180] Interpersonal Communication retrieved at: https://www.armyupress.army.mil/Journals/NCO-Journal/Archives/2017/October/Interpersonal-Communication/

The Current Solution: Set Boundaries

With expectations comes an ongoing tally of give and take. Who is giving more? Who is taking more? What is fair? What is unfair? This tally reflects the imbalance of power. Like Cicely and Liam, we rarely feel like the balance is in our favor. Some feel resentful that they're giving far more than they're getting in return. They're afraid of being taken advantage of. Others feel guilty or worried that they aren't able to give as much as the other person expects. They're afraid of being indebted.

To protect ourselves we set up boundaries. These communicate what we expect from others, including how we expect them to treat us and behave around us. We enforce our boundaries by establishing consequences to inflict on anyone that violates them. Our goal is to teach them to respect our boundaries better next time, thereby recorrecting the power imbalance. Some try to correct the perceived imbalance of power by exerting more power (e.g., taking your child's ear buds, rolling your eyes) or withholding support (e.g., refusing to drive, refusing to talk).

Why It's Not Solving the Problem

In order for boundaries to be effective, others must respect them. If they don't, our only recourse is to try to push them back with a consequence. This risks setting in motion a game of quid pro quo:

+ If they swear at me, then I'll give them detention.
+ If they don't pick up after themselves, then I'll take their phone away until they do.
+ If they do THAT to me, then I'll do THIS to them until I get my way.

Rather than teaching people to respect our boundaries, we get ourselves entwined in a power struggle. This is what happened with Cicily and Liam. The problem is, we're trying to control something that is not within our Circle of Control. Actually, several things. The other person must:

1. *Have a clear understanding of that boundary.* Let's say our boundary is "no swearing." For others to meet that boundary successfully they must know exactly what we consider swearing. Do we mean a handful of four-letter words or are we including words like "dang" and "darn." What about foreign words? Is it everyone or just kids? We may not even know what our boundary is until it's crossed.

2. *Remember the boundary.* What if every teacher has a different "no swearing" rule? It's a lot to expect that every child keeps track of the varying parameters of each rule. Even within our intimate relationships, it's difficult to remember the details of what we each need, especially since our boundaries are likely to change based on the situation, our mood, even the weather.

3. *Value the boundary.* Although swearing may be offensive and unacceptable to us, others may view them as a part of their daily vernacular. They may think that boundary is silly and even funny to cross. Authority figures tend to devalue, even ignore, the boundaries of their subordinates as well. Parents may enter their child's room without knocking or go through their stuff without asking. But turn it around and all hell breaks loose.

4. *Able to meet the boundary.* Keep in mind that not everyone will be able (or willing) to meet your needs. They may perceive them as unfair or counter to their own needs. They may have competing expectations of their own that you're not meeting and are trying to reset the imbalance of power. Remember Melissa

in Chapter 9 who expected her son to respect her demand to immediately put down his video game and do his homework without question? In other words, to stop doing what he loved, start doing something he disliked, and be happy about it. Her son resisted because his mom's expectations were counter to his need to have uninterrupted down time so he could de-stress. Regardless, she was upset because her boundary was crossed.

Even though there are many reasons why our boundaries may be violated, it still results in festering animosity, escalating conflict, mutual irritation, even irrational anger. If we feel like the victim, we may blame others for our circumstance and relinquish responsibility. The problem is, no matter how adamant we are about people respecting our boundaries, whether they do so or not will always remain outside our Circle of Control.

The TSC Solution: Relationship Reciprocity

Rather than expecting others to respect our limits, Relationship Reciprocity focuses on respecting our own limits (which *is* within our Circle of Control). By flipping the responsibility back on ourselves, Relationship Reciprocity safeguards us from being overwhelmed by the demands of others or disappointed by their responses.

How much am I willing to give?

We can decide how much we're willing to give to others and to the relationship–regardless of what we get (or don't get) in return. How much are we willing to give to our kids just because they're our kids? How much are we willing to give to work just because we take pride in what we do? No expectations. No price or consequences. We know we've hit our limit when we feel like we're about to pop. We may start to get irritated or feel like a walking doormat. Anything we do beyond that is setting us up to be disappointed and the other person to let us down.

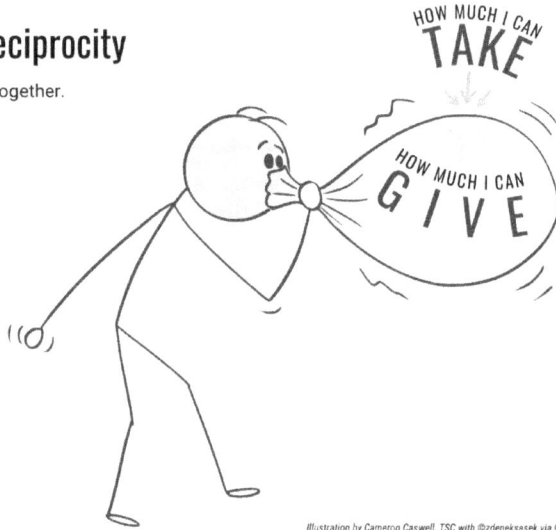

Relationship Reciprocity

PURPOSE: Protect when together.
HOW: Give + Take.

HOW MUCH I CAN **TAKE**

HOW MUCH I CAN **GIVE**

Illustration by Cameron Caswell, TSC with ©zdeneksasek via Canva.com

How much am I willing to take?

We can also decide what we can tolerate from someone else regardless of the other person's willingness to acknowledge or adapt to our needs. We know we've hit our limit when we feel deflated. We may get exhausted and nauseous after spending time with someone or notice that we're continually apologizing for no apparent reason just to try to appease them. Rather than getting upset at them for mistreating us or making us upset, we want to focus on what is in our control to enforce our limits.

One of our teen clients, Allisa, had been friends with Maria since preschool. They still talked on the phone a lot and would hang out on the weekends. But at school, Maria was rude to Allisa, especially in front of her new group of friends. Sometimes it was so bad that Allisa would hide in a bathroom stall to cry. Allisa finally confronted Maria about it. She told her how mean she was and said if she didn't stop being such a jerk, she wouldn't talk to her again. Maria shot back saying she'd be nicer if Allisa would stop being so annoying at school. They hadn't talked in weeks and now Maria was trying to hang out again. Although Allisa missed her, she was afraid Maria wouldn't change. She didn't know what to do.

We helped her identify four choices that were within her Circle of Control:

1. Stop being friends with Maria.
2. Continue being friends with Maria and tolerate her being mean to her at school.
3. Stay friends with Maria and stop doing whatever it was that annoyed Maria's friends and hope they stop being mean to her.
4. Stay friends with Maria, but define what treatment she was willing to tolerate. Rather than getting mad at Maria for disrespecting her limits (which was outside her control), she could respect her own limit by walking away (inside her control) or not approach her at school at all.

How much am I willing to risk?

At the beginning of the chapter we talked about our need for trust and respect. Neither can be obtained through coercion and control. We also cannot expect people to earn them based on merit. That's because none of us are immune to making mistakes and all it takes is one misstep for many to withdraw or withhold their trust and respect. Once lost, it's nearly impossible to gain back.

So how do we get it? The simple answer: you have to give it first. If you want more trust in a relationship, you have to give more trust. If you want more respect in a relationship, you have to be more respect-ful. This creates quite a conundrum for us humans. How do we trust someone that doesn't trust us? But that's exactly the point. How can we expect someone to trust us if we don't trust them? Someone has to go first. That requires that big, scary "V" word: Vulnerability. And we're still not guaranteed we're going to get it back. But without trying, we'll never know. Plus, the rewards are far greater than the risk. When we're more vulnerable, we're more likable[181] and able to form close relation-ships.[182] It's also one of the most powerful ways to earn genuine respect and trust.

With great power comes responsibility

Rather than having the *right* to respect and trust, the person with authority has the *responsibility* to be the first to give it. Rather than having the right to take from the other person, we must be the ones that ensure we are fostering connection, leading with curiosity, and generous with compassion.

Let's go back to Cicily and Liam. Because Cicily was the authority figure, she felt it was her right to demand Liam to respect her. Because he didn't, she justified not respecting him back. That's not how it works. If Cicily wants Liam to respect her, the only thing she can do is start by showing him respect. That's how he learns what respect looks like. And only when he feels respected by the person in power will he trust them enough to be vulnerable and respect them. Same goes for Melissa and

---

[181] Hodgins (1996)

[182] Hopwood et. al. (2021)

her son. She wanted him to respect her, but she clearly didn't have any respect for his needs. When both boys tried to assert their limits, they were immediately shut down, labeled as disrespectful and slapped with consequences. We simply can't expect children to trust and respect adults if adults don't show them trust and respect first. Fortunately, when we focus more on what we have control over and less on what we don't, we can account for the needs of others without sacrificing our own.

The power of no

"No" is one of the first words we learn as a child, yet one of the most difficult words to say as an adult. We've been groomed to be people pleasers since childhood when saying "no" was perceived as defiance and met with disapproval.

As adults, we still carry that fear of disappointing others and will agree to things we don't want to just to avoid it.[183] We may not want to risk upsetting someone or being perceived as selfish and mean. However, saying "no" helps us respect our limits, stick to our priorities, and feel in control of our lives. If you're still uncomfortable saying "no," remember that you're always saying no to something. So, before you say "yes" to something, first identify what you're now saying "no" to.

---

[183] https://ecommons.cornell.edu/bitstream/handle/1813/74812/Bohns1_Misunderstanding_our_influence.pdf;jsessionid=34E1889FF25CD08EA193888E012A83B5?sequence=1

Getting the N.A.C. of It

Step 1: NOTICE you need relationship reciprocity

Notice how you feel when you hit your limit. You may feel like you're about to explode if you've hit the max of what you can give. You may feel like you're about to implode when you've hit the max of how much you can take. Remember to notice with curiosity, not criticism.

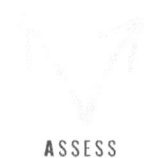

NOTICE

Step 2: ASSESS if it's helpful or hurtful.

A simple way to determine if a limitation is helpful or hurtful is to look at our Circle of Control. Good indicators that you're relying on someone else to keep our limits are words like "You" and "Should":

ASSESS

YOU should know better.

YOU should be more grateful.

YOU should trust me.

YOU shouldn't say that.

YOU shouldn't do that.

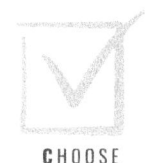

Step 3: CHOOSE what to do next

When we notice someone is impinging on your limits, it's up to us to decide what to do.

CHOOSE

Choice #1: Stick with it

You have the choice to continue doing exactly what you've been doing, and you can already predict the outcome. If the outcome is what you want, great. If it's not, just realize that by choosing not to change, there is little chance the outcome will either.

If it's a relationship with a child or family member, you may not be willing to dissolve it no matter how hurtful it gets, we understand that. If it's a relationship between a colleague, co-parent, or teammate, you may not have the option to sever it. In these cases, it's important to acknowledge that we can't force someone to meet our expectations any more than they can force us to meet theirs. We encourage you to try reframing it instead.

Choice #2: Neutralize it

Rr   Escape Space

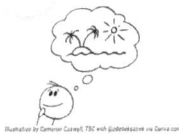

Illustration by Cameron Casey, TSC with @johnlukas116 via Canva.com

Though it's best to have your eyes closed for this Rapid Reset, we understand that may not feel safe. No problem. Just look at the ground or find a focal point in the room instead. Envision a space that brings you a sense of peace and calm. Some examples are the beach, hiking in the woods, watching a sunset, etc. Tap into as many senses as you can in that space. Think about how the air might feel against your skin, what sounds you might hear, and what you might see, taste, or smell. Sit in that space and absorb those sensory feelings as much as you can. Open your eyes or reengage when you're feeling calm.

Choice #3: Reframe it

In order to respect our own limitations, we must first get as clear as we can on what they are. Ask, "How much am I willing to give regardless of what I get in return?" "How much am I willing to tolerate regardless of the other person's willingness to acknowledge or adapt to my needs? Then get clear about what you can do to maintain your limits that's within your Circle of Control. For example, "You can be angry, but I'm not going to tolerate being called a %^&#! I'm going to walk away now. When you're open to talking with me without calling me that, I'm here." Remember, you can be respectful and firm at the same time.

The Biggest Takeaways

		How do I know I've reached my limit?	What is in my control to respect that limit?
	GIVE		
	TAKE		

1. Authority doesn't give us the right to respect and trust. Authority gives us the responsibility to give it.
2. Determine how much you are willing to give and take regardless of what you get in return.
3. We can't expect others to respect our limits. It is our responsibility to respect them instead.

CHAPTER 11

~

Compassionate Communication

"Never attribute to malice that which can be adequately explained by misunderstanding."

–Hanlon's Razor[184]

When you send a message (through actions or words), are you aware of how others have received it? Do they interpret it as an act of love or an act of control? Do they see it as an act of encouragement or a passive aggressive put down? Do they believe you're really concerned or laying a guilt trip? If their response is not what we were hoping for, chances are, they didn't receive it the way we wanted them to.

The Problem: Building Barriers

Miscommunication is the root of most problems. That's no secret. A lot can go wrong when we communicate which creates barriers to connection.

---

[184] https://hbr.org/2019/11/why-groups-struggle-to-solve-problems-together

Let's take a look at some common ways people create these barriers:

	Barrier	Outcome
1	Make an inaccurate assumption.	Feel misunderstood or misrepresented.
2	Use our own cultural norms to interpret a message.	May not account for differing tones, expressions, body language, etc.
3	Weave in irrelevant information.	Confuse the message and appear incompetent.
4	Over-explain with too many details.	Use up too much time and mental energy.
5	Send a message full of underlying contempt.	Appear to be mean, rude, or distrustful.
6	Let emotions overtake us (exhaustion, hunger, stress).	Disconnect from others.
7	Omit significant information from the message.	Lose trust in the source.
8	Speak on behalf of others without getting their input.	Feel undervalued.
9	Use only one communication method.	Alienate people.
10	Disengage out of fear of being misunderstood.	Increases isolation.

Let's consider a scenario with Rinaldo, a 16-year-old who lives with his grandmother (his guardian). Rinaldo's curfew is 11:00 p.m.. While watching a movie at a friend's house one night, he realizes that the movie will go longer than expected. It's 10:50

p.m., and Grandma gets a call from Rinaldo. "Hi, Grandma, can I come home at 11:30 p.m. tonight?" Grandma, rousing from sleep, asks, "How come?" His explanation made sense to Grandma. "I guess so" with a sleepy, edgy tone. "Ok, thanks, Grandma. See you soon." Rinaldo had an uneasy feeling when he hung up the phone. He thought, *Why did she give me so much attitude? I called to ask permission and was being responsible.* When he came home and passed his grandma on the stairs, he felt defensive. When his grandma asked, "How was the movie?" Rinaldo responded, "Fine", which had an edgy tone. His grandma thought, *Why did he give me so much attitude? I appreciated his call and gave him permission to stay.* She went to bed feeling defensive.

What went wrong? The breakdown occurred when both Rinaldo and his grandmother each had contempt in their responses after making an inaccurate assumption that the other was being insulting; both of them were wrong.

With the limitless options of how these two might wake up in the morning and interact, there will likely be some level of conflict. Maybe Grandma will ask Rinaldo to come down for breakfast but because she's holding on to last night's negative feeling, she's easily frustrated when he doesn't immediately comply. Rinaldo, still ruminating from having to come home to tension after a fun night out with his friends, avoids coming downstairs altogether.

Communicating without context

When we don't have a clear idea of the message someone is sending us (miscommunication), we make assumptions to interpret its meaning; that's where it gets dangerous. Relying on only ourselves to decipher someone else's intention without context only adds confusion. To compensate, we try to communicate more (e.g., ask more questions, send more texts) or resort to ineffective strategies like demanding, nagging, pleading, yelling, and raging. This is when one or both of us climbs the Ladder of Conflict, and the underlying message, or intention, gets lost in the abyss of emotion. Once this happens, we've created a divide, and we displace our frustration on the other person for not receiving our message the way we wanted them to.

Without context, someone may perceive us as being rude, dishonest, or judgmental. It feels like an attack on their character, and they disengage. If we're not careful with our intentionality, they hear messages that devalue them like "You're unimportant" or "You're not worth it" or "You're incompetent," and this crushes their spirit. This is especially true when authority figures (e.g., teachers, parents, coaches) speak down to kids. Even if our intention is "good," if they perceive it's bad, then there's a disconnect.

On the flip side, when we have uncertainty about someone else's intention, we default to making assumptions. This is dangerous because we might be wrong and may shut someone out unnecessarily. We lose opportunities for meaningful relationships that would enhance our lives as a result, and eventually risk eroding our connections altogether.

Why It Matters

Meaningful relationships are essential to our health and well-being. When we don't pay closer attention to our interactions, it puts us at a higher risk for offending someone or feeling offended by someone, causing unnecessary tension and conflict.[185] Since this dilemma creates divide and causes some people to spiral into serious mental health issues, we need to have more awareness of how we're showing up. We're shutting down the opportunity for connection when we put up these barriers and sometimes devalue people, and/or ourselves, in the process.

---

[185] Colombo, M. W. (2004). Family literacy nights and other home-school connections. Educational Leadership, 61(8), 48-51.

We disengage when misunderstood

When our message is misconstrued, it can create long-term issues for both sides involved. If our tone is interpreted as being mean, for example, we feel misunderstood and misrepresented. The response feels unjustified. We get defensive and end up forgetting what the initial purpose of the communication was in the first place, leading to hurt feelings. One incident, such as with Rinaldo and his grandmother, might dissolve overnight on its own, though when this pattern occurs over time, the relationship can deteriorate. Trust is lost. We disengage, and we may give up trying because the recurrent painful feelings aren't worth it anymore.

Others disengage when they misunderstand us

Conversely, we create barriers when the other person doesn't believe we have their best interest at heart, or we've let them down too many times. Even if we mean well, if the other person doesn't believe that, we lose them. Rather than cultivating more connection, we foster more fear, anxiety, and insecurity. Nobody's thriving in this climate. We saw how this dynamic can affect family relationships with Rinaldo and his grandmother. Now, let's take a look at how it's corroding our school communities.

The impact on school climate

How educators communicate either enhances connectedness or rouses tension based on the underlying feelings they evoke. We know students feed off that energy, so when data shows that poor communication is a leading cause of work-related stress and a catalyst for quitting,[186] we

---

[186]https://www.globenewswire.com/news-release/2019/03/20/1757785/0/en/Dynamic-Signal-Study-Finds-U-S-Workforce-Stressed-and-Ready-to-Quit-Compounding-Concerns-From-Tight-Labor-Market-and-Possible-Economic-Downturn.html

want to make revisions there. Because effective communication is the glue that builds trust and security, it is essential to retaining staff and maintaining morale. When there is a breakdown, it can be felt within the whole school community.

The impact on parent engagement

Though schools are trying to make connections with parents, parents are reporting dissatisfaction[187] or feeling isolated.[188] Both want what's best for the child. The problem is, they don't always agree on what that is or how to achieve it. Even if they do, when poorly communicated, it creates misunderstanding and builds conflict, which gives them little to no hope for resolution. It's a lose-lose situation. Say nothing, nothing gets addressed. Speak up, things may get more difficult.

On the other hand, when parents and educators are in touch and have positive interactions, everyone benefits. Students have increased motivation, improved academic performance, and better behavior.[189] Students also develop a strong sense of belonging and have more engagement.[190] [191] When we consider the impact of the spillover effect (chapter 2), improving communication among parents and school staff will reduce stress everywhere.

[187] Noel (2015)

[188] NSPRA (2006)

[189] Khan Alamgir , Dr Salahuddin Khan, Syed Zia-Ul-Islam, & Manzoor Khan (2017). "Communication Skills of a Teacher and Its Role in the Development of the Students' Academic Success." Journal of Education and Practice

[190] Dinu, 2015

[191] Richmond Virginia, P. (1990). "Communication in the classroom: power and motivation." communication education

The impact on youth mental health

We want kids feeling secure enough to approach the adults in their world. Having that lifeline is critical to their well-being and affects their school experience. Their test scores and grades improve and their attendance and participation increases. Their social skills, self-esteem, and emotional control all strengthen,[192] [193] [194] so there are clearly positive outcomes when parents and school staff build connections for their sake. Clear, respectful communication is the culprit when this isn't happening. When adults are not getting along, our children feel it, and may not know who to trust.

Kids are always watching us. Since they are impressionable and will emulate our actions, we need to be mindful about what those are. If adults are not proficient communicators, then children who learn from them will not be either. We want our children to grow up to be advocates for themselves and get along with others well, so we need to show them how to do it.

The Current Solution: Improve Communication

There are numerous communication tools to help us engage in the communication process (think "I" statements...). We're taught to use filters or break down barriers. We learn about how these roadblocks keep us from getting our message across the way we intend it to come across. We understand that non-verbal language sends stronger messages than our words do, so we learn to change our posture, align our gestures and expressions, and get feedback to check for accuracy. This process gets complicated.

---

[192] National Center for Education Statistics (2019)
[193] Henderson, A.T. & Berla, N. (1994)
[194] American Federation of educators (2007)

Why It's Not Solving the Problem

There are plenty of strategies to help us become better communicators, though when there is conflict, these are difficult to access or use in a pinch. Sometimes there are just too many steps to follow. Racing thoughts, feelings, body language cues and words that get flung around while we're trying to concentrate on the takeaway message, all while getting our own point across, is tricky. Just envisioning this elicits discomfort.

Complexity breeds confusion

Like active listening, the traditional communication process is powerful and can make a positive impact when used properly. However, it ends up being inauthentic because we're trying so hard to get all the steps right and in order. We misuse the skills often as a means to get what we want, which comes off as manipulation. We seem, or *are*, dishonest, which creates disconnect. Here, we lose trust in the *person*.

One misstep can create a breakdown in the whole operation. If it's ineffective, we lose trust in the *process*. Even when we are willing to continue communicating, everyone needs to have proficiency in whichever model they're using, and if not, it may be used improperly. When this dynamic happens regularly, it causes cynicism. Regardless of who's to blame, when any or all of us are entering a conversation defensively or with resentment, no one wins. Even when a problem gets resolved, the affliction creates further divide.

Blame it on the brain

Even though the rational, more civilized part of our brain has more effective tools to make sense of someone's message and participate in the communication process, we usually let our primitive brain lead. This reactivity causes us to get easily frustrated and misinformed.

Who is this really about?

Another reason for a breakdown is that we're more focused on ourselves and getting our point across. We try to convince the other person that we're right or that our message is more important than theirs. We focus more on being *understood*, rather than *understanding* someone else. We get so caught up in this internal demand that we forget to check if we're solving the problem. We certainly aren't creating a connection, and if we don't care about either of these, there's no forward movement.

In our schools, communication among all three pillars interchangeably needs to be meaningful and genuine. If even one person is seething in anger, feeling rejected, or withdrawing, we're missing the mark.

The TSC Solution: Compassionate Communication

In order to have more clear and meaningful communication, we need to focus only on two simple, yet critical, pieces:

1. SEND: Send your message with a *respectful intention*, and
2. RECEIVE: Ensure it's *received* as intended.

Compassionate Communication

PURPOSE: Connect together.
HOW: Send + Receive

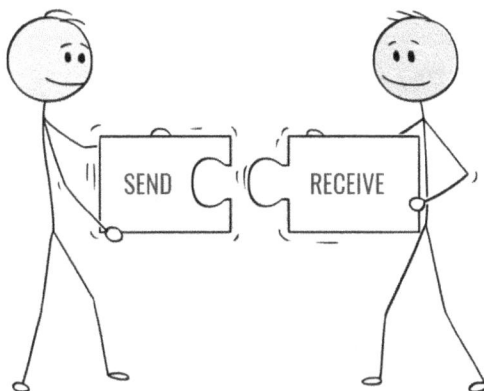

SEND RECEIVE

Illustration by Cameron Caswell, TSC with ©zdeneksasek via Canva.com

Let's consider a situation with our client Mia:

> Mia was especially heartbroken about her dream of a close-knit family slipping away. She expressed that she felt like she was the only one making an effort to stay close. She planned family dinners and movie nights, gave her kids lots of hugs and said "I love you" several times a day. Mia said her children acted like they wanted nothing to do with her. They avoided her and made snide remarks when passing by. Mia felt like most of their anger was directed at her and couldn't understand where it was coming from.

Mia's intention was respectful...so what's the problem? Though Mia's intention was kind in nature, her kids weren't receiving it that way. Because they perceived her attempts of "love" as "controlling," there was contention with every "I love you" or call to dinner. When Mia learned to communicate with her kids and altered how she sent "love" the way her kids would receive it, she subsequently drew the family back together.

When these two pieces of Compassionate Communication (send + receive) work together interchangeably, we produce a welcoming atmosphere where people can freely engage.

Getting the N.A.C. of It

NOTICE

Step 1: NOTICE you need Compassionate Communication Notice how the other person is responding to you. If they're responding in a way that does not match what you were intending, just notice that. Remember to notice with curiosity, not criticism.

ASSESS

Step 2: ASSESS if it's helpful or hurtful

If people are warm, welcoming, and accepting of you, the way you're communicating is likely helpful.

If people are not responding the way you're intending or are hostile, annoyed, or avoidant with you, then it's likely hurtful.

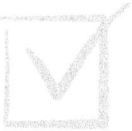

CHOOSE

Step 3: CHOOSE what to do next

Choice #1: Stick with it

You have the choice to continue doing exactly what you've been doing, and you can already predict the outcome. If the outcome is what you want, great. If it's not, just realize that by choosing not to change, there is little chance the outcome will either.

Choice #2: Neutralize it

If we feel ourselves getting frustrated because they're not responding the way we were hoping, we can neutralize our emotions with Rapid Resets.

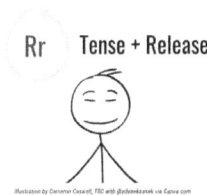

Rr   Tense + Release

Illustration by Cameron Caswell, TBC with @adeekeamek via Canva.com

Notice where your tension is and tense up those surrounding muscles as tightly as you can for 5-10 seconds. Then release them. For example, if your jaw is tense, press your tongue to the roof of your mouth and hold. Release. You can do this with your fists, shoulders, or wherever you tension.

Choice #3 Reframe it

We want to approach communication as a cooperative activity. It's something we do together, not to or at each other. If we're feeling like our intention is not understood when sending our message, you may notice a shift in behavior or expressive language, arguing, or avoidance. You can think, "Is my intention respectful?" or "Are they feeling respected?" If the answer is unclear, we need to reframe. Use this tool to help:

It's important to make sure your intention is respectful and is being received that way. Minimize translation errors with these simple questions throughout the conversation. Check in to confirm. We build connection when we consistently show up to people with respectful intentions. Use Compassionate Communication to continue to do that.

	I know my intention is respectful* when...	I know my intention is disrespectful when...
SEND		
RECEIVE		

* Although we encourage you to start with respect, you can also insert other intentions (e.g. loving, kind, assertive, etc.)

Illustration by Cameron Caswell, TSC with ©zdeneksasek via Canva.com

The Biggest Takeaways

1. We want our children to grow up to be advocates for themselves and get along with others well, so we need to show them how to do it.

2. In our schools, communication among all three pillars inter-changeably needs to be meaningful and genuine.

3. If we use a respectful intention and check that it's being received correctly, we build connection.

CHAPTER 12

∼

Collaborative Resolution

*"We can't solve problems by using the same kind of
thinking we used when we created them."*

−Albert Einstein

As a society, we've become more polarized than ever.[195] Our intolerance for listening to other perspectives or interacting with people who hold dissimilar views is growing dramatically in both size and intensity.[196] [197] This is reflected in our personal relationships, too.

---

[195] http://www.gallup.com/poll/197828/record-high-americans-perceive-nation-divided.aspx

[196] Iyengar S., Lelkes Y., Levendusky M., Malhotra N., Westwood S.J. The origins and consequences of affective polarization in the United States. Ann Rev Polit Sci. 2019;22:129–146.

[197] Pew Research Center. 2017. The Partisan Divide on Political Values Grows Even Wider. Available at https://www.people-press.org/2017/10/05/the-partisan-divide-on-political-values-grows-even-wider/

The Problem: Polarization

There is a heavy reliance on top-down decision making,[198] from implementing district-wide reforms to setting classroom rules. Educators depend on the principal to make decisions which impact their work conditions and practices. Parents must entrust their children's school to create a safe learning environment, and students rely on parents and educators to create a place they feel accepted and belong.

Power imbalance

If people in power make decisions without gathering sufficient context or getting buy-in, when it trickles down, it increases distrust and a sense of unfairness. It decreases commitment and enthusiasm. It also makes people suspicious about the intention behind decisions. We often assume that decisions are based mainly on the self-interest of the decision maker with little or no regard to our personal interest or needs.

We heard from one middle school Vice Principal that educators were asked to use a supplementary learning program in which the district had purchased for them. The educators had already integrated a different program into their lesson plans, so they disregarded the request. Administration insisted that they stop using the old program and use the new one they had purchased. Educators were frustrated that they were being forced to relearn a new system and redo their entire lesson plans on top of all the excessive record keeping and planning they already had to do. Even worse, the new system was cumbersome and restrictive. Several of the educators decided to pitch in and buy the program they liked using their own money. However, when they called the

198

company to purchase it, they were told that their administrators ordered them to ban educators from their district. Educators consequently felt angry and defeated.

This dynamic occurs in our personal and family lives too. Consider this typical exchange at home with a parent and child.

Parent: "Time to do your homework."

Child: "OK." Five minutes later, the child hasn't moved.

Parent: "What are you doing?! I told you to go do your homework."

Child: "I know! I just want to finish this game first." Five minutes later, the child still hasn't moved.

Parent: "That's enough. Go do your homework NOW!"

Child: "Stop nagging me. It's not even due until next week."

Parent: "That's it!" [fed up with being disrespected] "I'm taking your phone until you learn to talk to me respectfully."

Child: "You're the worst parent ever."

These exchanges are exhausting and rarely end with even one person happy, let alone both.

Why It Matters

The issues burdening our school communities today (e.g., disciplinary policies, standardized testing, and bullying) continue to grow. We experience similar polarization at home when it comes to discipline, technology use, and academic performance, just to name a few. Each new challenge creates an opportunity to initiate positive change and improve practices and increase connection. However, despite our best efforts and intentions, our attempts fall short due to a lack of trust.[199] That's

---

[199] https://www.sciencedaily.com/releases/2008/08/080827164035.htm

because imposing solutions onto people without fully understanding their problem or hearing their perspective is not only ineffective, but it can also have seriously negative consequences.

The district allotted a healthy budget to spend on classroom supplies. Dr. Callen, an elementary school administrator, decided to thoughtfully purchase a year's supply of pencils for every classroom teacher, thinking they would appreciate the gesture. Afterall, SO many students lose or forget their pencils on a daily basis, and it's a common complaint overheard in the staff room. Dr. Callen had the pencils delivered to the staff room. Imagine Dr. Callen's surprise when some teachers groaned when she announced these were what she spent the funding on. What went wrong?

Dr. Callen had an enormous heart for teachers and genuinely wanted to solve one of their persistent problems. However, she missed the mark because some teachers already spent their own money on pencils and didn't need them. If Dr. Callen had asked them what they needed, rather than assume everyone needed the same thing, teachers would have felt more appreciated.

The erosion of trust

As trust erodes, so does confidence in one another. Educators question district initiatives. Parents question school directives. Students question rules and consequences. Employees get distracted with office politics. Before we know it, we have sparked little fires of contention everywhere. This leaves little time to find and implement long-lasting, equitable solutions. On the other hand, when we work in an environment which fosters high levels of trust we are less stressed, more productive, and more engaged.[200] We all perform better in this climate and experience wellness more often.

The Current Solution: Problem-Solving Models

A popular approach to solving problems on a systems level is implementing a collaborative problem-solving strategy. The goal with this is to work together to achieve shared success. There are a plethora of models that can be used to facilitate this: heuristics, methods, processes, activities, and of course, plain ol' trial-and-error. We are taught to use these models in our personal lives too. With so many options to choose from, it seems like problems should be easier to solve. So why do we still have conflict?

Why It's Not Solving the Problem

Even small problems elicit roadblocks when trying to come up with a solution. We discussed how complicated the communication process can be in Chapter 11, so is the process of problem-solving. Our assumptions, biases, and cultural perceptions get in the way during a complex thought process.[201] This is especially difficult when more than two people enter into the equation where more assumptions come into play.[202]

They don't address deep-seeded distrust

The nature of these problems also evokes deep emotions. Though people usually are well-intentioned and want to do better, they may feel

---

[200] Zak, Paul, "The Neuroscience of Trust," Harvard Business Review, 2017. https://hbr.org/2017/01/the-neuroscience-of-trust

[201] https://www.frontiersin.org/articles/10.3389/feduc.2020.538202/full

[202] https://hbr.org/2019/11/why-groups-struggle-to-solve-problems-together

stuck in painful feelings of the past. While collaboration strategies can work, they fall short when the underlying problem isn't accounted for: distrust. No matter how effective a tool is, if we don't find a way to overcome distrust, our collaborative effort is bound to fail. Without trust, we feel compelled to act in our own best interest rather than in the general good. If we enter the collaborative process with a preconceived goal or solution in mind, we can use the tool to manipulate the outcome, much like we discussed in the communication process (Chapter 11).

They don't account for power imbalance

When there is an authority role in the dynamic, there may be an imbalance of power. They can use their power to swing the results in their favor, forcing the less influential to concede. Those who are more emphatic (and often extreme), may become fixated on convincing others to agree to what they believe is right, even if the process uncovers flaws in their rationale and strengths in another's.[203] The process ends up being a charade that may appear collaborative on the outside, but in reality opposing sides may show up ready to fight rather than open their mind to resolve a problem. Working in harmony towards a common goal may be challenging in this dynamic.

When collaboration becomes too difficult, we're likely to quit altogether or revert to our individual silos to come up with our own solutions. In theory, this sounds easier and more empowering, but when our solutions become fragmented and possibly conflicting, we end up back where we started—putting out little fires everywhere.

---

[203] Stavrakakis Y. Paradoxes of polarization: democracy's inherent division and the (anti-) populist challenge. Am Behav Sci. 2018;62:43–58.

The TSC Solution: Collaborative Resolution

Because systematic processes of stages and steps allow more room to err,[204] we need a simple tool to resolve complex issues. It also must level the playing field and build a mutual sense of security and trust. To do this, we pruned the process down to focus on just one thing: What we each need THE MOST. We call this Collaborative Resolution.

The beauty is in the simplicity. Rather than getting caught up in the process, we are able to get laser focused on needs and how to meet those needs. We start by identifying the ONE thing each person needs the most by asking these three basic questions:

1. What is the ONE thing you need most?
2. What is the ONE thing I need the most?
3. How do we help each other get what we need?

Collaborative Resolution

PURPOSE: Resolve together.

HOW: The One Thing

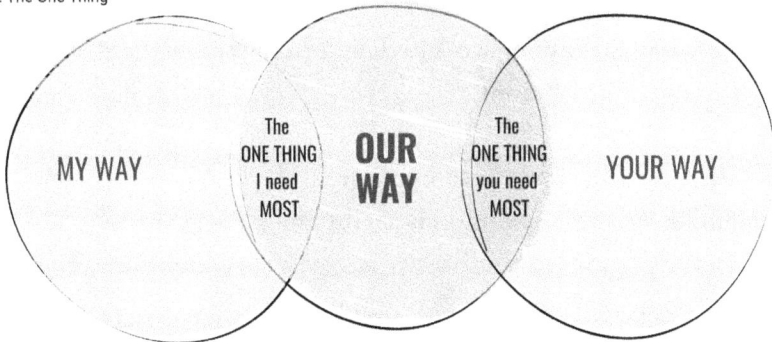

MY WAY | The ONE THING I need MOST | OUR WAY | The ONE THING you need MOST | YOUR WAY

Illustration by Cameron Caswell, TSC

---

[204] https://hbr.org/2019/11/why-groups-struggle-to-solve-problems-together

A balance of trust and power

- Because we are able to communicate what we need the most, we feel empowered and valued. When people feel like their voice is heard and their needs are met, they no longer have to be forced to comply.

- Because it prompts us to self-select our top priority, it ensures a satisfactory solution. No one is left feeling like their needs weren't accounted for.

- Because our need must be met in order for someone else's need to be met, it builds a sense of security and trust. We now are free to direct our energy and focus on the solution rather than using it to defend and protect our position.

- Because everyone's needs, regardless of authority or persistence, are treated with equal importance, it ensures a more equitable solution. When everyone's needs are met, we build trust, strengthen relationships, and set the entire group up to thrive.[205] [206]

Let's replay the homework exchange from early in the chapter using Collaborative Resolution:

Parent: "Time to do your homework."
Child: "OK." Five minutes later, the child hasn't moved.
Parent: "I noticed you haven't started your homework yet. What's going on?"
Child: "I'm exhausted and just want to chill."
Parent: "I understand. I'm exhausted after a long day, too. What's your plan?"

---

[205] https://www.princeton.edu/news/2021/12/09/political-polarization-and-its-echo-chambers-surprising-new-cross-disciplinary

[206] https://files.eric.ed.gov/fulltext/EJ1067214.pdf

Child: "My homework isn't due until 6th period tomorrow. It's only going to take me about 10 minutes and I have a study hall in the morning."

Parent: "The ONE thing I need is to know you're not going to forget. How can you help me with that?"

Child: "What if I text you when I finish it tomorrow?"

Parent: "That works. I'll text you during Study Hall if I don't hear from you, just in case you forget to text me."

The ONE thing the parent needed was to know their child had a plan to do their homework and wasn't just blowing it off. The ONE thing the child needed was to have autonomy over their homework. Rather than trying to make their child comply with their solution (get it done immediately) they were open to finding a solution that met both their needs. This allowed their child to own their homework while still gaining reassurance that they were being accountable.

Imagine what we could do if administrators, educators, parents, and students collaborated this way to find solutions for common issues like classroom disruption, academic discrepancies, and poor mental health. How many problems could we solve if we stepped out of the blame game, came together as allies rather than adversaries, and focused on Collaborative Resolution instead?

Getting the N.A.C. of It

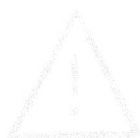

Step 1: NOTICE you need Collaborative Resolution
Notice when you are confronted with a problem. Remember to notice with curiosity, not criticism.

NOTICE

Step 2: ASSESS if it's helpful or hurtful

ASSESS

When we enter into disagreements with a preconceived solution or an expected outcome, our participation in the collaborative effort is likely hurtful. This mindset squashes curiosity, innovation, and the opportunity to discover an equitable solution. When we are committed to finding a solution that equally addresses the ONE need of the other person and our own, our collaborative effort is likely helpful.

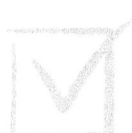

Step 3: CHOOSE what to do next

Choice #1: Stick with it

CHOOSE

You have the choice to continue doing exactly what you've been doing, and you can already predict the outcome. If the outcome is what you want, great. If it's not, just realize that by choosing not to change, there is little chance the outcome will either.

Choice #2: Neutralize it

When you're struggling to resist engaging in a cyclical argument, it helps to neutralize your emotions with Rapid Resets.

Rr   Alphabet Soup

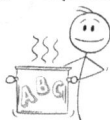

For the Alphabet Soup Rapid Reset, start naming types of food from A to Z. A-apple, B-banana, C-carrot, etc. Stop when you're feeling calm. Go through it again if you need more time to settle.

Choice #3: Reframe it

Start by identifying the ONE thing you each need the MOST. This ensures you are focusing on everyone's top priority. Acknowledge that everyone believes as strongly in their opinion as you do in yours. Everyone wants their needs met as much as you do.

Once we've identified the ONE thing we both need the MOST, we are ready to find a solution that helps us each get what we need.

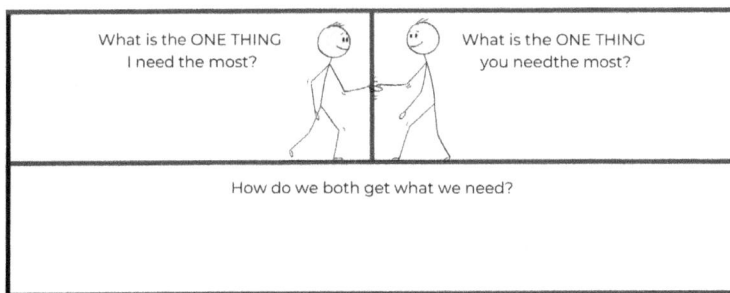

What is the ONE THING I need the most?

What is the ONE THING you needthe most?

How do we both get what we need?

Illustration by Cameron Caswell, TSC with gardenekzazek via Canva.com

We worked with a mom, Roberta, who was irritated that her 17-year-old son refused to drive. They fought over it daily. She had done everything she could think of to make her son drive: yelled at him, pleaded with him, bribed him with money, and took all his devices away. Nothing worked. She was over it. She chalked it up to her son being difficult.

We asked Roberta to identify the ONE thing she needed the MOST. She scoffed and said, "For my son to drive already." What she identified as a need was actually her preconceived solution to the problem. Because she was determined to get the outcome she expected, she wasn't open to collaborating. This resulted in regular heated battles with her son.

We asked her, "What is the ONE thing you need that is resolved by him driving?" It turned out that Roberta wanted to attend a weekly group that conflicted with her son's soccer practice. She had been looking forward to her teen being able to drive himself so she would finally be free to go. However, her son was terrified that he was going to get into an accident, so was resistant to get behind the wheel. Bingo.

The ONE thing her son needed the most was to get to practice. The ONE thing the mom needed the most was to attend the weekly group. Now she was ready to figure out with her son how he could get to practice, and she could still make her meeting. This is Collaborative Resolution in action.

In order to adapt to life's challenges in the space of others, it's important to have the flexibility to integrate the needs of others into our own. Instead of challenging one another as adversaries, we learn to face challenges together as allies. This removes unnecessary ego, drama, and defensiveness, which only serve to distract us from finding a solution and sap us of our time, energy, and rationality. Only when we let go of our need to win, do we open ourselves up to seeing, understanding, and resolving the underlying problem and discovering the best outcome for everyone.

The Big Takeaways

1. With Collaborative Resolution, everyone has an equal voice because everyone matters: administrators, educators, staff, parents, and students.

2. What is the ONE thing I need the most? What is the ONE thing you need the most? How do we help each other get what we need?

3. Collaborative Resolution provides a safe space for people with differing values and views to come together with the goal of finding an equitable solution.

PART III

~

Leading a Thriving School Community

The TSC framework fosters the development of healthy, supportive relationships which leads to increased student academic achievement, improved behavior, and well-being.[207] Since feeling safe with others is probably the "single most important aspect of mental health,"[208] building a culture of connection is a crucial step to establishing a thriving school community. Leaders have the power to initiate this culture of support, and because your staff carries a heavy load, they deserve some attention. Students need to like their school, want to be there, and feel a strong sense of belonging, so do educators.

---

[207] Konald et al., 2018

[208] Sapiens, Cooperation 15:50

~

CHAPTER 13

How To Get Started

"The journey of a thousand miles begins with a single step."

—Lao Tzu

Because cooperation is the central theme of human advancement and is the key to reaching a common goal, we need to work together towards a thriving school community. Create a buzz, devise your plan, and announce it to staff highlighting your priority to put their mental health first. They'll thank you for it, and you'll protect your human capital. While developing your action plan, remember to:

+ Simplify programming so it's easy to get started.
+ Integrate skills into everyday practice.
+ Prevent problems from occurring in the first place.

How Administrators Can Use the TSC Framework

With your school team, you'll use data you've already collected to create a snapshot of the current state of mental health in your building and aim to fill disparity gaps.

Cover Equity and Inclusion Initiatives

The TSC framework is an essential piece to your equity and inclusion plan. Data shows consequential academic inequities among marginalized groups[209] saturated with educators who may have limited experience working with them.[210] With improved academic and wellness outcomes for kids of all backgrounds when the nine skills are embedded in their school culture, the school becomes a place of respite. Everyone has a chance to thrive here. You'll break down barriers so that there is a constant healthy exchange among people who advocate for themselves and each other and resolve their differences with dignity.

Take Care of Your Teaching Staff

You need buy-in anytime you introduce a new program or initiative. Since teachers are the first to benefit from this plan, they'll likely buy-in. Teachers have told us that they want to improve their skills and appreciate the opportunity to get their needs met. This is particularly true when it is based on their specific requests. For example, if educators are struggling with avoidant students, they can learn how to effectively respond to their anxious students using Allo skills. If your team notices an influx of teacher absences, they would benefit from learning more about Auto skills. Because the nine skills provide solutions to a wide variety of problems, you can use them to resolve those disparity gaps you find in your data.

---

[209] (Clotfelter, 2004; Orfield, Ee, Frankenberg, & Siegel-Hawley, 2016; Owens, Reardon, & Jencks, 2016; Reardon & Owens, 2014); https://journals.sagepub.com/doi/full/10.3102/0002831219868182

[210] Leath, Mathews, Harrison, & Chavous, 2019; https://journals.sagepub.com/doi/full/10.3102/0002831219868182#bibr79-0002831219868182

Invest in Parents

Chances are, you already have initiatives to involve parents in your schools. Often these sit idle, though, because there isn't a plan which entices parents or is simple enough to set in motion. What a great opportunity this is to maximize your parent engagement efforts! You can provide parents with the same valuable tools you're giving school staff so all adults are working in tandem to support your students.

How Educators Can Use the TSC Framework

Though the primary role of an educator isn't to deal with student mental health issues, they *are* in this position at times. They invest in the well-being of students well beyond academics which makes them an integral part of the mental health team. There's no need to be consumed with the high demands of this profession, however. We're giving educators permission to look after themselves and release the overwhelm.

Practical tools and strategies are sprinkled throughout this book and can have an immediate effect on staff and student wellness. Teachers will use tools like the Circle of Control to determine if an outcome is something they can influence or not, or when they find themselves in an argument, they can visualize the Ladder of Conflict to determine if they want to climb it or not. Teachers can also use these tools with students. For example, when students approach them with a dilemma, they can pull out the Path of Possibilities, modeling and showing the student how to take ownership in the choices they are making. The TSC framework will provide them with practical tools and strategies to infuse mental health practices into their day which works for every grade level. With easy-to-implement tools, educators will conserve their energy, integrity, and sanity so they can focus on the most important things in their work and home life starting from a calmer baseline.

The Biggest Takeaways

1. Your school community is desperate for change. Provide them with assurance that mental health is a top priority by putting an action plan in place.
2. Fill disparity gaps using the data you've already collected to make changes to the current state of your school's mental health.
3. Customize experiences for educators based on their voice and need; they'll have buy-in and will feel valued.

CHAPTER 14

～

Future Vision

"The key to realizing a dream is to focus not on success but significance—and then even the small steps and little victories along your path will take on greater meaning."

–Oprah Winfrey

Attendance, report cards, test scores, graduation rates, college and career readiness[211] are all impacted by poor mental health; initiating change now will begin improving these areas in our education system. We know that until all members of your school community are functioning well,[212] students will not perform optimally.

With growing rates of serious mental illnesses and increasing youth suicide rates,[213] we need to act fast. Teacher retention is also a problem we need to quickly mitigate. The system will implode without educators functioning well, or without them there at all. Whether they're leaving your building or exiting the profession, too much is at

---

[211] Aspen Institute (2019)
[212] White House Fact Sheet (2022)
[213] Walrath, 2015; Education Development Center, 2022

stake if we don't do something different now. Leveraging our schools to improve youth wellness will ensure a faster outcome.

Making a Culture Shift

Underdeveloped countries are successfully using some of these paralleled strategies that are "cheap to operate" and "easy to scale,"[214] so the proof of a simplistic yet comprehensive solution in how we address mental health exists. Since so many youth suffer in silence, even though they are surrounded by plenty of compassionate adults, schools are positioned to make significant impacts. Widespread, incremental shifts we make here will have a transformative effect on youth mental health long-term, spilling into the way we function as a whole society.

Initiating a powerful wave of cultural change will ensure longevity. When all members of the community are participating and working together, rather than in silos, we operate more harmoniously. This culture of connectedness cascades into other areas of life and becomes ingrained in our daily vernacular. Since all nine skills are adaptable and appropriate for all age groups and across all settings, we can have a profound effect on future generations.

All three pillars (staff, students, and parents) have the same level of importance in the thriving school community. Because we equip all of them with the nine essential skills and share in an immersive cultural experience where the skills are constantly modeled and reinforced, we have sustainability, even when changes occur. As concerns about our students' mental health continue to rise, the parent/school partnership creates a "critical, complementary team" to benefit students,[215] so

[214] https://www.vox.com/the-highlight/23402638/mental-health-psychiatrist-shortage-community-care-africa

[215] https://healthpayerintelligence.com/news/cvs-health-how-educators-parents-factor-into-adolescent-mental-health

schools have a vested interest. Because students also build proficiency in the nine skills, they become more self-reliant in managing their own problems and well equipped to adapt and cope. They will learn the skills we all wish we were taught at a young age which would have helped us function better, get in less trouble, make better decisions, get along with others and be more compassionate.

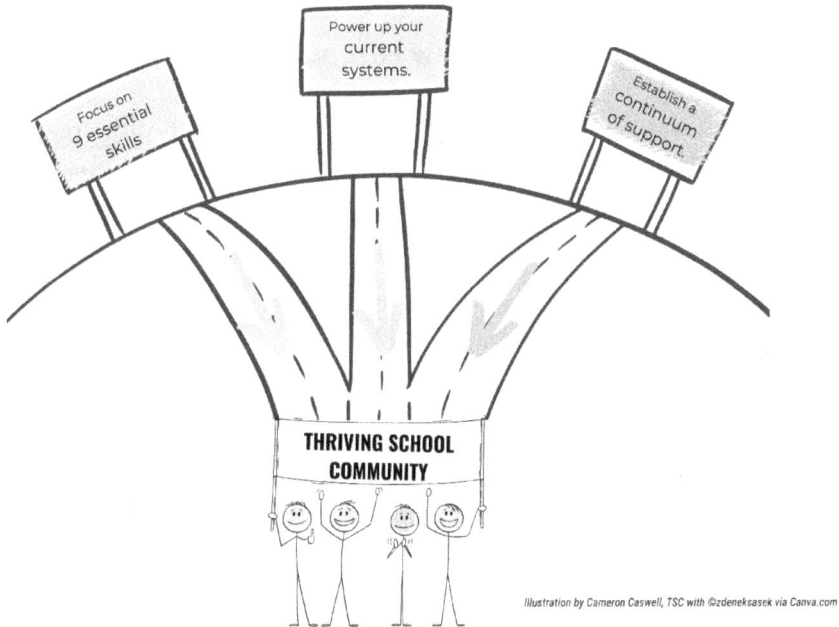

Illustration by Cameron Caswell, TSC with ©zdeneksasek via Canva.com

Adapting the TSC Framework

Though we target schools in this book, the TSC framework is adaptable to other facets of society. Because we get down to the fundamentals of functioning well as human beings, organizations and corporations who want to create their own thriving culture will benefit, too.

New Teacher Education Programs

Mental health training is scarce[216] in university teacher programs. If we equip aspiring teachers in our education programs with these nine skills, we give them vital tools to use when they enter their practicums. By the time they enter their own classrooms, they'll be proficient and can pass the skills on to their students.

A Proactive Approach for New Parents

Prevention is a key aspect in averting another mental health crisis in the future. We need to reach kids early. Those considering parenthood and new parents with young children are perfect candidates for early intervention. Before their children enter our school systems, we'd like to better equip them, too. Training new parents will help kids thrive well before they show up to our schools.

The Biggest Takeaways

1. Unless the adults in your school community are functioning well, students will not perform optimally.
2. When all members of the community are participating and working together, rather than in silos, we operate more harmoniously.
3. Schools are positioned to make widespread shifts and have a transformative effect on youth mental health long-term, spilling into the way we function as a whole society.

---

[216] (Fazel et al., 2014, p. 390).

CHAPTER 15

~

The Final Takeaway

"The opposite of love is not hate; it's indifference."

–Dr. Eva Olsson, LLD (Hon), Holocaust Survivor

What side of history do you want to be on? What legacy do you wish to leave behind, and what major social shifts do you want to be a part of? If your heart leans toward improving the youth mental health crisis, we encourage you to take action now.

Our action or inaction can be equally powerful. We learned a compelling message from Kevin Hines, a man who jumped off the Golden Gate Bridge and lived to tell about it. He was in such a deep state of despair and believed suicide was the only way to release the pain of living. However, after he jumped, he instantly regretted it. He emphasized that we must acknowledge others because it might be the one and only chance we have to save their life. Kevin told us that he was willing people to just ask him if he was OK on his way to the bridge because he wouldn't have jumped if they had done so.

Schools have the power to save lives. So many kids sit in our buildings feeling alone, are battling an affliction, or are contemplating suicide and don't know what to do next. Apathy and avoidance are damaging. Because we don't know what to do, we further isolate them by leaving them to struggle in silence. Not all stories lead to suicide, of course, though inevitably there are plenty of kids who wish someone would reach out to them, see them, listen to them, smile at them, even just notice their existence. [217]

Those who hold the power to influence the trajectory of young people's lives need the crucial skills to get it right. We envision change in every school community throughout the country so we can give our children the future they deserve. That future depends on the collective actions we all take together. Today's youths are relying on us to set them up to thrive, so the sooner we start, the sooner they will benefit.

[217] Carr, E.W., Reece, A., Kellerman, G.R., Robichaux, A. (2019). The Value of Belonging at Work. Harvard Business Review. Retrieved at: https://hbr.org/2019/12/the-value-of-belonging-at-work

Appendix A

Rapid Resets

Hand to Heart

Rr Hand to Heart

Illustration by Cameron Caswell, TSC with @zajeroksazek via Canva.com

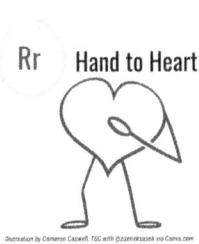

This is a therapeutic technique used with variations such as putting a hand to your forehead or your stomach or using your left versus right hand. The effects are there with any of these, so let's keep it simple and just place one of your hands over your heart. Sit, stand, or lay down comfortably. You can close your eyes or find a focal point in the room to look at such as the floor or a picture. The goal is to attune to your body responses when feeling even the slightest distress so you can protect yourself from spiraling too deeply into despair, which is difficult to move out of. Notice where you're feeling strain, and picture untangling that for relief. Try to bring your breath to an in-through-the-nose and out-through-the-mouth in a slow, steady pattern. With your hand, gently but firmly still placed over your heart, pay attention to anywhere you need to unravel discomfort. You can add in some reassuring words to remind yourself of your strengths. Tell yourself that you deserve freedom from being stuck in this moment and will move out of it when you're ready to take that step. Just like you did as an infant, you have the ability to self-soothe.

Thumb Drum

Rr   Thumb Drum

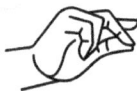

Illustration by Cameron Caswell, TSC with @iamAbc via Canva.com

This is a great time to use if you need to raise your energy, such as when you're feeling unmotivated or sluggish, or lower your energy, such as when you're feeling antsy or anxious. You can do this without anyone knowing about it, which is why we love Thumb Drum for those who want to be discrete.

Take either hand and bring each of your fingers to your thumb. Change the pressure as needed, depending on whether you need to get extra energy out (add pressure) or whether you need to go from chaos to calm (lighten the pressure). You can also quicken the pace moving from finger to finger if you need to increase your energy level. You can slow down the pace if you need to decrease your energy level.

Finger Thumb Switch

Rr   Finger-Thumb Switch

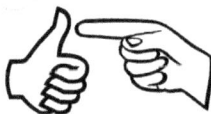

Illustration by Cameron Caswell, TSC

Put your left thumb up (like you're giving a "thumbs up"). Stick out your right pointer finger towards your left thumb. In a simultaneous motion, quickly switch to opposite positions - stick out your left finger at your right thumb. This will take practice, but eventually, you'll train your brain to do it in a swift, seamless motion. This is great to do before starting a task where you need to be laser focused like learning a complex topic, taking a test, playing a game.

Stop Sign

Picture a stop sign in your head. Envision yourself tracing the outline of the stop sign and see the word STOP grow from small to large.

Rr Stop Sign

Continue repeating this process until you no longer feel the urge to take an impulsive action.

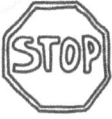

Illustration by Cameron Caswell, TEC with @itsandiconapro via Canva.com

\Inhale, Exhale

Rr Inhale/Exhale

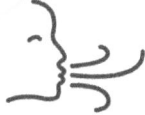

Take one deep breath in through your nose as slowly as you can. Now exhale through your mouth as slowly as you can. Repeat until you feel calm.

Illustration by Cameron Caswell, TEC with @bombjunny11 via Canva.com

Climb Down the Ladder

Rr Ladder of Conflict

When you're aware that you are feeling discomfort, picture yourself freezing on the bottom rung of the ladder, and slowly climb down. If you've already climbed up, it's ok. Picture yourself freezing there and slowing climbing back down. This visual reminder will help alter your physical and emotional state, bringing you back to *calm*.

Illustration by Cameron Caswell, TEC

Escape Space

Rr Escape Space

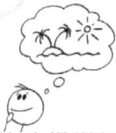

Though it's best to have your eyes closed for this Rapid Reset, we understand that may not feel safe. No problem. Just look at the ground or find a focal point in the room instead. Envision a space that brings you a sense of peace and calm. Some examples are the beach, hiking in

Illustration by Cameron Caswell, TEC with @izdesellzasiek via Canva.com

the woods, watching a sunset, etc. Tap into as many senses as you can in that space. Think about how the air might feel against your skin, what sounds you might hear, and what you might see, taste, or smell. Sit in that space and absorb those sensory feelings as much as you can. Open your eyes or reengage when you're feeling calm.

Tense + Release

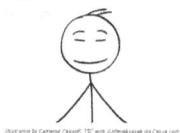

Rr Tense + Release

Notice where your tension is and tense up those surrounding muscles as tightly as you can for 5-10 seconds. Then release them. For example, if your jaw is tense, press your tongue to the roof of your mouth and hold. Release. You can do this with your fists, shoulders, or wherever you tension.

Alphabet Soup

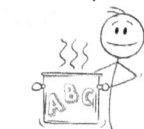

Rr Alphabet Soup

For the Alphabet Soup Rapid Reset, start naming types of food from A to Z. A-apple, B-banana, C-carrot, etc. Stop when you're feeling calm. Go through it again if you need more time to settle.

References

Adams, K. (2021, December 13). Why investing in SEL now may be the key to an equitable future. EdSurge. https://www.edsurge.com/news/2021-12-13-why-investing-in-sel-now-may-be-the-key-to-an-equitable-future

American Psychological Association. (2022). APA dictionary of psychology. https://dictionary.apa.org/behavioral-health

Arango, C., Díaz-Caneja, C. M., McGorry, P. D., Rapoport, J., Sommer, I. E., Vorstman, J. A., McDaid, D., Marín, O., Serrano-Drozdowskyj, E., Freedman, R., & Carpenter, W. (2018). Preventive strategies for mental health. The lancet. Psychiatry, 5(7), 591–604. https://doi.org/10.1016/S2215-0366(18)30057-9

Armstrong, L. E., Ganio, M. S., & Casa, D. J., et al. (2012). Mild dehydration affects mood in healthy young women. J Nutrition, 142(2), 382-388. doi:10.3945/jn.111.142000

Aspen Institute. (2019). From a nation at risk to a nation at hope: Recommendations from the National Commission on Social, Emotional, & Academic Development Centers for Disease Control (CDC). YRBSS data summary & trends. Center for Disease Control and Prevention. https://eric.ed.gov/?q=source%3A%22Aspen+Institute%22&id=ED606337

Atkins, M. S., Hoagwood, K. E., Kutash, K., & Seidman, E. (2010). Toward the integration of education and mental health in schools. Administration and policy in mental health, 37(1-2), 40–47. https://doi.org/10.1007/s10488-010-0299-7

Ayish, K. & Deveci, T. (2019). Student perceptions of responsibility for their own learning and for supporting peers' learning in a project-based learning environment. International Journal of Teaching and Learning in Higher Education, 31(2). 221-237.

Buttner, A. (2021, April 19). The teacher shortage, 2021 edition. [Podcast]. Frontline Education. https://www.frontlineeducation.com/blog/teacher-shortage-2021/

CASEL. (2022). Our history. About. CASEL. https://casel.org/about-us/our-history/

CASEL. (2020). A reintroduction to SEL: CASEL's definition and framework. [Youtube Video]. https://www.youtube.com/watch?v=0N_Y34tjQm8

Caviness, V. S., Jr, Kennedy, D. N., Richelme, C., Rademacher, J., & Filipek, P. A. (1996). The human brain age 7-11 years: A volumetric analysis based on magnetic resonance images. Cerebral Cortex (New York, N.Y. : 1991), 6(5), 726–736. https://doi.org/10.1093/cercor/6.5.726

CDC. (2022). Suicide Prevention Resource for Action: A compilation of the best available evidence. Atlanta, GA: National Center for Injury Prevention and Control, Centers for Disease Control and Prevention. https://www.cdc.gov/suicide/pdf/preventionresource.pdf

Chamberlin, J. (2009, January). Schools expand mental health care. Monitor on Psychology, 40(1). http://www.apa.org/monitor/2009/01/school-clinics

Committee for Children. (2019, January 7). Record high demand for social-emotional learning in US schools. [Blog]. Committee for Children blog. https://www.cfchildren.org/blog/2019/01/record-high-demand-for-social-emotional-learning-in-us-schools/

Darling-Hammond, L., Flook, L., Cook-Harvey, C., Barron, B. & Osher, D. (2020). Implications for educational practice of the science of learning and development. Applied Developmental Science, 24(2), 97-140, DOI: 10.1080/10888691.2018.1537791

Darling-Hammond, L.,Hernández, L. E., Schachner, A., Plasencia, S., Cantor, P., Theokas, C., & Tijerina, E. (2021, September). Design principles for schools putting the science of learning and development

into action. Learning Institute and Turnaround for Children. https://
k12.designprinciples.org/sites/default/files/SoLD_Design_Principles_
REPORT.pdf

Durkheim, E. (1951). Suicide: A study in sociology (2nd ed.). Routledge.
https://doi.org/10.4324/9780203994320

Edutopia. (2011, October 6). Social and emotional learning: A short history
teaching the soft skills, traditionally associated with conflict resolution
and character education, has evolved from being considered "wishy-
washy" to being an integral part of educating the whole child. https://
www.edutopia.org/social-emotional-learning-history

Fazel, M., Hoagwood, K., Stephan, S., & Ford, T. (2014). Mental health
interventions in schools 1: Mental health interventions in schools in
high-income countries. The lancet. Psychiatry, 1(5), 377–387. https://
doi.org/10.1016/S2215-0366(14)70312-8

Forte, G., Morelli, M., & Casagrande, M. (2021). Heart rate variability and
decision-making: Autonomic responses in making decisions. Brain
sciences, 11(2), 243. https://doi.org/10.3390/brainsci11020243

Gallup. (2014). State of America's Schools: The Path to Winning
Again in Education. https://www.ncbi.nlm.nih.gov/pmc/articles/
PMC6350815/#R21

GBAO Strategies. (2021, January 31). Poll results: Stress and burnout
pose threat of educator shortages. National Education Association
(NEA). https://www.nea.org/sites/default/files/2022-02/NEA%20
Member%20COVID-19%20Survey%20Summary.pdf

Hari, J. (2015, June). Everything you think you know about addiction
is wrong. [Youtube Video]. TED Global London. https://
www.ted.com/talks/johann_hari_everything_you_think_you_
know_about_addiction_is_wrong

Mozes, A. (2022, March 14). Mental health of America's children only
getting worse. University of Rochester Medical Center. Health
Encyclopedia https://www.urmc.rochester.edu/encyclopedia/content.
aspx?contenttypeid=6&contentid= 1656915363

Herman, K. C., Hickman-Rosa, J., & Reinke, W. M. (2018). Empirically
derived profiles of teacher stress, burnout, self-efficacy, and coping and

associated student outcomes. Journal of Positive Behavior Interventions, 20(2), 90–100. https://files.eric.ed.gov/fulltext/EJ1173521.pdf

Horowitz, J. M. & Graf, N. (2019, February 20). Most U.S. teens see anxiety and depression as a major problem among their peers: For boys and girls, day-to-day experiences and future aspirations vary in key ways. Pew Research Center. https://www.pewresearch.org/social- trends/2019/02/20/most-u-s-teens-see-anxiety-and-depression-as-a-major-problem-among-their-peers/#academics-are-at-forefront-of-the-pressures-teen-face

Jennings, P. A., & Greenberg, M. T. (2009). The prosocial classroom: Teacher social and emotional competence in relation to student and classroom outcomes. Review of Educational Research, 79(1), 491–525.

Jimenez, E. C. (2021). Impact of mental health and stress level of educators to learning Resource Development." Shanlax International Journal of Education, 9(2), 1-11. DOI: https://doi.org/10.34293/ education. v9i2.3702

Jotkoff, E. (2022, February 1). NEA survey: Massive staff shortages in schools leading to educator burnout; alarming number of educators indicating they plan to leave profession. National Education Association (NEA). https://www.nea.org/about-nea/media-center/ press-releases/ nea-survey-massive-staff-shortages-schools-leading-educator

Kamenetz, A. (2022, February 1). More than half of educators are looking for the exits, a poll says. NPR. https://www.npr. org/2022/02/01/1076943883/educators-quitting-burnout

Konold, T., Cornell, D., Jia, Y., & Malone, M. (2018). School climate, student engagement, and academic achievement: A latent variable, multilevel multi-Informant examination. AERA Open. https://doi. org/10.1177/2332858418815661

Lever, N., Mathis, E., & Mayworm, A. (2017). School mMental health is not just for students: Why teacher and school staff wellness matters. Rep Emotional Behavior Disorders Youth, 17(1), 6–12. https://www. ncbi.nlm.nih.gov/pmc/articles/PMC6350815/pdf/nihms-982083.pdf

Lebrun-Harris, L. A., Ghandour, R.M., Kogan, M. D., & Warren, M. D. (2022). Five-year trends in US children's health and well-being, 2016-2020. JAMA Pediatrics. E1-E11. doi:10.1001/ jamapediatrics.2022.0056

Maloy, A. F. (2020, November 12). Distance learning is straining parent-teacher relationships. The Washington Post. https://www.washingtonpost.com/lifestyle/2020/11/12/ parent-teacher-relationships-covid/

McCormick, J., & Barnett, K. (2011). educators' attributions for stress and their relationships with burnout. International Journal of Educational Management, 25(3), 278–293

McGraw Hill. (2021, September 27). New K–12 survey: Social and emotional learning gains awareness and prioritization amid COVID-19 pandemic. https://www.mheducation.com/news-media/press-releases/ social-and-emotional-learning-survey-2021.html

Mental Health First Aid International. (2012). Youth mental health First Aid USA: For adults assisting young people. National Council for Behavioral Health.

Miron, O., Yu, K.-H., Wilf-Miron, R., & Kohane, I. S. (2019). Suicide rates among adolescents and young adults in the United States, 2000-2017. JAMA: Journal of the American Medical Association, 321(23), 2362–2364. https://doi.org/10.1001/jama.2019.5054

Morrison, N. (2021, December 24). Stopping the great teacher resignation will be education's big challenge for 2022. Forbes. https://www. forbes.com/sites/nickmorrison/2021/12/24/stopping-the-great-teacher-resignation-will-be-educations-big-challenge-for-2022/?sh=b84f073157cd

Neece, C. L., Green, S. A., & Baker, B. L. (2012). Parenting stress and child behavior problems: a transactional relationship across time. American journal on intellectual and developmental disabilities, 117(1), 48–66. https://doi.org/10.1352/1944-7558-117.1.48

Noel, A., Stark, P., & Redford, J. (2016, June). Parent and family involvement in education, from the National Household Education Surveys Program of 2012. National Center for Education Statistics. https://nces.ed.gov/pubs2013/2013028rev.pdf

Owens, M. T., & Tanner, K. D. (2017). Teaching as Brain Changing: Exploring Connections between Neuroscience and Innovative Teaching. CBE life sciences education, 16(2), fe2. https://doi.org/10.1187/cbe.17-01-0005

Pianta, R., Downer, J., & Hamre, B. (2016). Quality in early education classrooms: Definitions, gaps, and systems. Future of Education, 26(2), 19-137. https://files.eric.ed.gov/fulltext/ EJ1118551.pdf

Sparks, D., Ralph, J., & Malkus, N. (2015, December). Stats in brief: Public school teacher autonomy in the classroom across school years 2003–04, 2007–08, and 2011–12. U.S. Department of Education-National Center for Education Statistics. https://nces.ed.gov/pubs2015/2015089.pdf

Quaglia Institute for Student Aspirations, Teacher Voice and Aspirations International Center, and Corwin Press. (2016). School Voice Report. Quaglia School Voice; Corwin Press. https://quagliainstitute.org/dmsView/School_Voice_Report_2016

Riess, T. (2017). The science of empathy. Journal of Patient Experience, 4(2), 74-77. https://www.ncbi.nlm.nih.gov/pmc/articles/PMC5513638/pdf/10.1177_2374373517699267.pdf

Robert Wood Johnson Foundation. (2017, September). Teacher stress and health: Effects on educators, students and schools. The Pennsylvania State University. https://drive.google.com/file/d/18faM1M0_k9jFv9bOT0-pzAFz6cYgGCLU/view

Sharot, T., Shiner, T., Brown, A. C., Fan, J., & Dolan, R. J. (2009). Dopamine enhances expectation of pleasure in humans. Current Biology, 19(24), 2077–2080. https://doi.org/10.1016/j.cub.2009.10.025

Steiner, E. D. & Woo, A. (2021). Job-related stress threatens the teacher supply: Key findings from the 2021 State of the U.S. Teacher Survey. RAND Corporation. https://www.rand.org/content/dam/rand/pubs/research_reports/RRA1100/RRA1108-1/RAND_RRA1108-1.pdf

The U.S. Surgeon General's Advisory. (2021). Protecting youth mental health. U.S. Department of Health & Human Services. https://www.

hhs.gov/sites/default/files/surgeon-general-youth-mental-health-advisory.pdf

Thompson, D. (2019, June 18). U.S. youth suicide rate reaches 20-year high. U.S. News & World Report. https://www.usnews.com/news/health-news/articles/2019-06-18/us-youth-suicide-rate-reaches-20-year-high

Tierney, J. (2011, August 7). Do you suffer from decision fatigue? The New York Times Magazine. https://www.nytimes.com/2011/08/21/magazine/do-you-suffer-from-decision-fatigue.html?_r=0

Umberson, D., Crosnoe, R., & Reczek, C. (2010). Social relationships and health behavior across life course. Annual Review of Sociology, 36, 139–157. https://doi.org/10.1146/annurev-soc-070308-120011

Umberson, D., & Montez, J. K. (2010). Social relationships and health: A flashpoint for health policy. Journal of Health and Social Behavior, 51, S54–S66. https://doi.org/10.1177/0022146510383501

University of Oxford. (2020, June 5). The neurobiology of social distance: why loneliness may be the biggest threat to survival. University of Oxford: News and Events. https://www.ox.ac.uk/news/2020-06-05-neurobiology-social-distance-why-loneliness-may-be-biggest-threat-survival

van Woerkom, M. & Meyers, M.C. (2019). Strengthening personal growth: The effects of a strengths intervention on personal growth initiative. Journal of Occupational and Organizational Psychology. 92(1). 98-121. https://doi.org/10.1111/joop.12240

Watts, W. D., & Short, A. P. (1990). Teacher drug use: A response to occupational stress. Journal of Drug Education, 20(1), 47–65. https://doi.org/10.2190/XWW0-7FBH-FXVB-2K3C

Wallman, M. & O'Matz, B. (2022). Violent kids take over Florida's classrooms, and they have the law on their side. South Florida Sun Sentinel. https://projects.sun-sentinel.com/teenage-time-bombs/how-schools-manage-violent-kids

Widnall, E., Price, A., Trompetter, H., & Dunn, B. D. (2020). Routine cognitive behavioural therapy for anxiety and depression is more effective at repairing symptoms of psychopathology than enhancing wellbeing. Cognitive Therapy and Research, 44(1), 28–39. https://doi. org/10.1007/s10608-019-10041-y

Witvliet, C. v., Ludwig, T. E., & VanderLaan, K. L. (2011). Granting forgiveness or harboring grudges: Implications for emotion, physiology, and health. Psychological Science, 12(2), 117-123. https://greatergood. berkeley.edu/images/uploads/VanOyenWitvliet -GrantingForgiveness. pdf

Woolf, N. (2022). CASEL releases new definition of SEL: What you need to know. [Blog Post]. Panorama. https://www.panoramaed.com/blog/ casel-new-definition-of-sel-what-you-need-to-know

Yard, E., Radhakrishnan, L. Ballestors, M. F. , et al. (2021). Emergency department visits for suspected suicide attempts among persons ages 12-25 years before and during the COVID-19 pandemic -United States, January 201-May 2021. MMR Morb Mortal Wkly, 70, 888-894. DOI: http://dx.doi.org/10.15585/mmwr.mm7024e1

Yettick, H. (2018, September 28). Demand for social-emotional learning products and services is high and expected to grow: Vast majority of K-12 school districts have invested in SEL or will do so over the coming year, survey finds. Education Week - Edweek Market Brief. https:// marketbrief.edweek.org/exclusive-data/sel/

About the Authors

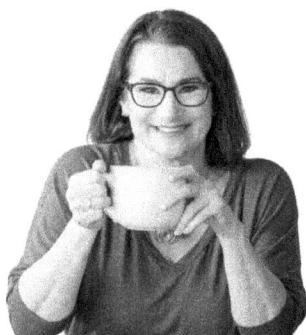

Cameron (**Dr. Cam**) **Caswell**, PhD, the "teen translator," is an adolescent psychologist, family success coach, and co-creator of *Thriving School Community*, a revolutionary program designed for schools to improve student, staff, and parent well-being. For over two decades, she has been helping parents build strong, positive relationships with their teens through improved communication, connection, and understanding. Dr. Cam is a TEDx speaker, host of the Parenting Teens with Dr. Cam podcast, co-creator of the "I Am Enough" teen 12-week workshop, author of Power Phrases for Parents: Teen Edition, and co-author of Improving School Mental Health: The Thriving School Community Solution. Dr. Cam is the mom of a teen too, so she not only talks the talk, she walks the walk! Connect with Dr. Cam at: drcam@thrivingschool.org

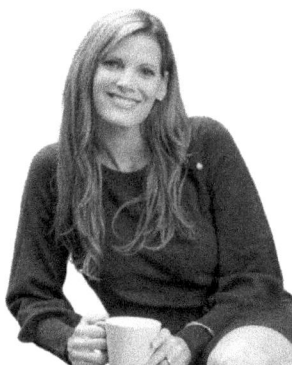

Charle Peck is the is the co-creator of *Thriving School Community*, a revolutionary program designed for schools to improve student and staff mental health. With over twenty years of education and mental health leadership experience, she has the unique lens of both a certified teacher and a licensed therapist. Charle holds an MS in Education and an MS in Social Work. Her role as a high school teacher coupled with her clinical work with children and families in crisis gives her incredible insight into solving youth mental health problems stemming from our schools. She is the co-author of *Improving School Mental Health: The Thriving School Community Solution* and a global keynote speaker delivering powerful messages of hope to educators. Connect with Charle at: charle@thrivingschool.org

More from ConnectEDD Publishing

Since 2015, ConnectEDD has worked to transform education by empowering educators to become better-equipped to teach, learn, and lead. What started as a small company designed to provide professional learning events for educators has grown to include a variety of services to help educators and administrators address essential challenges. ConnectEDD offers instructional and leadership coaching, professional development workshops focusing on a variety of educational topics, a roster of nationally recognized educator associates who possess hands-on knowledge and experience, educational conferences custom-designed to meet the specific needs of schools, districts, and state/national organizations, and ongoing, personalized support, both virtually and onsite. In 2020, ConnectEDD expanded to include publishing services designed to provide busy educators with books and resources consisting of practical information on a wide variety of teaching, learning, and leadership topics. Please visit us online at connecteddpublishing.com or contact us at: info@connecteddpublishing.com

Recent Publications:

Live Your Excellence: Action Guide by Jimmy Casas
Culturize: Action Guide by Jimmy Casas
Daily Inspiration for Educators: Positive Thoughts for Every Day of the Year by Jimmy Casas
Eyes on Culture: Multiply Excellence in Your School by Emily Paschall
Pause. Breathe. Flourish. Living Your Best Life as an Educator by William D. Parker

L.E.A.R.N.E.R. Finding the True, Good, and Beautiful in Education by Marita Diffenbaugh

Educator Reflection Tips Volume II: Refining Our Practice by Jami Fowler-White

Handle With Care: Managing Difficult Situations in Schools with Dignity and Respect by Jimmy Casas and Joy Kelly

Disruptive Thinking: Preparing Learners for Their Future by Eric Sheninger

Permission to be Great: Increasing Engagement in Your School by Dan Butler

Daily Inspiration for Educators: Positive Thoughts for Every Day of the Year, Volume II by Jimmy Casas

The 6 Literacy Levers: Creating a Community of Readers by Brad Gustafson

The Educator's ATLAS: Your Roadmap to Engagement by Weston Kieschnick

In This Season: Words for the Heart by Todd Nesloney, LaNesha Tabb, Tanner Olson, and Alice Lee

Leading with a Humble Heart: A 40-Day Devotional for Leaders by Zac Bauermaster

Recalibrate the Culture: Our Why…Our Work…Our Values by Jimmy Casas

Creating Curious Classrooms: The Beauty of Questions by Emma Chiappetta

Crafting the Culture: 45 Reflections on What Matters Most by Joe Sanfelippo and Jeffrey Zoul

ConnectEDD
PUBLISHING

www.ingramcontent.com/pod-product-compliance
Lightning Source LLC
Chambersburg PA
CBHW070107030426
42335CB00016B/2044